Genetics for Pulmonologists

The Remedica Genetics for... Series
Genetics for Cardiologists
Genetics for Dermatologists
Genetics for Hematologists
Genetics for Oncologists
Genetics for Ophthalmologists
Genetics for Orthopedic Surgeons
Genetics for Pulmonologists
Genetics for Rheumatologists

Published by the REMEDICA Group
REMEDICA Publishing Ltd, 32–38 Osnaburgh Street, London, NW1 3ND, UK
REMEDICA Inc, Tri-State International Center, Building 25, Suite 150, Lincolnshire, IL 60069, USA
E-mail: books@remedica.com
www.remedica.com
Publisher: Andrew Ward
In-house editor: Charissa Deane
Design: REGRAPHICA, London, UK

ISBN 1 901346 45 5
British Library Cataloguing-in Publication Data
A catalogue record for this book is available from the British Library

Printed at Ajanta Offset & Packagings Limited, India.

Genetics for Pulmonologists
The molecular genetic basis of pulmonary disorders

Jordan Prutkin
CRTP Fellow
Pulmonary-Critical Care Medicine Branch
National Heart, Lung, and Blood Institute
National Institutes of Health
Bethesda, MD

Joel Moss
Chief
Pulmonary-Critical Care Medicine Branch
National Heart, Lung, and Blood Institute
National Institutes of Health
Bethesda, MD

Series editor:
Eli Hatchwell
Investigator
Cold Spring Harbor Laboratory

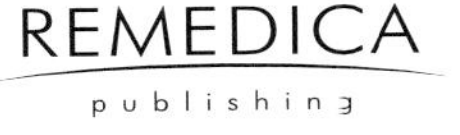

LONDON • CHICAGO

Introduction to Genetics for... series

Medicine is changing. The revolution in molecular genetics has fundamentally altered our notions of disease etiology and classification, and promises novel therapeutic interventions. Standard diagnostic approaches to disease focused entirely on clinical features and relatively crude clinical diagnostic tests. Little account was traditionally taken of possible familial influences in disease.

The rapidity of the genetics revolution has left many physicians behind, particularly those whose medical education largely preceded its birth. Even for those who might have been aware of molecular genetics and its possible impact, the field was often viewed as highly specialist and not necessarily relevant to everyday clinical practice. Furthermore, while genetic disorders were viewed as representing a small minority of the total clinical load, it is now becoming clear that the opposite is true: few clinical conditions are totally without some genetic influence.

The physician will soon need to be as familiar with genetic testing as he/she is with routine hematology and biochemistry analysis. While rapid and routine testing in molecular genetics is still an evolving field, in many situations such tests are already routine and represent essential adjuncts to clinical diagnosis (a good example is cystic fibrosis).

This series of monographs is intended to bring specialists up to date in molecular genetics, both generally and also in very specific ways that are relevant to the given specialty. The aims are generally two-fold:

(i) to set the relevant specialty in the context of the new genetics in general and more specifically

(ii) to allow the specialist, with little experience of genetics or its nomenclature, an entry into the world of genetic testing as it pertains to his/her specialty

These monographs are not intended as comprehensive accounts of each specialty — such reference texts are already available. Emphasis has been placed on those disorders with a strong genetic etiology and, in particular, those for which diagnostic testing is available.

The glossary is designed as a general introduction to molecular genetics and its language.

The revolution in genetics has been paralleled in recent years by the information revolution. The two complement each other, and the World Wide Web is a rich source of information about genetics. The following sites are highly recommended as sources of information:

1. PubMed. Free on-line database of medical literature.
   http://www.ncbi.nlm.nih.gov/PubMed/

2. NCBI. Main entry to genome databases and other information about the human genome project.
   http://www.ncbi.nlm.nih.gov/

3. OMIM. On line inheritance in Man. The On-line version of McKusick's catalogue of Mendelian Disorders. Excellent links to PubMed and other databases.
   http://www.ncbi.nlm.nih.gov/omim/

4. Mutation database, Cardiff.
   http://www.uwcm.ac.uk/uwcm/mg/hgmd0.html

Eli Hatchwell
Cold Spring Harbor Laboratory

Preface

This is an exciting time in molecular medicine. With the completion of the initial characterization of the human genome, we have the first blueprint for the construction of a human being. The functions of only a small fraction of the approximately 30 000 genes are known, and a rapid explosion in gene discoveries is now expected. The next step will be from genomics to proteomics, the description of all the proteins made from the genetic information. The sequence of a gene conveys information about the primary structure of the encoded protein or proteins and provides some clues regarding mechanisms for regulation of their synthesis. The tertiary structure of the protein, post-translational modifications, interactions with other molecules, intra- or extracellular localization, and functions must still be elucidated.

A great advance in the study of genetic diseases occurred in 1989 with cloning of the gene that, when mutated, causes cystic fibrosis. The positional cloning strategy used to identify the cystic fibrosis transmembrane conductance regulator (CFTR) became a model in the search for other disease-causing genes. Since that time, knowledge of the molecular functioning of CFTR has certainly grown, but understanding how this defect in electrolyte transport leads to colonization by bacteria and inflammation in the lung remains elusive.

The discovery of individual variations within genes, known as polymorphisms, and their relationship to diseases will be an important area of research. Polymorphisms in several candidate genes are already being investigated for their relationship with asthma. Other research is examining how specific polymorphisms modify the clinical course of various diseases. The relationship between genes encoding molecules involved in inflammation and the response to infectious agents is an engaging area of investigation.

In this book, we attempt to provide an overview of lung diseases for which the genetic defect has been defined as of June 2001. It is not intended to be complete, but rather to be an easy-to-use manual, with concise reviews of genetic diseases that a pulmonologist might encounter. For more detailed information, the Online Mendelian Inheritance of Man (http://www.ncbi.nlm.nih.gov/omim), created and maintained by Victor A. McKusick, M.D. and his colleagues at the Johns Hopkins University (Baltimore, MD) and developed by the National Center for Biotechnology Information, National Institutes of Health (Bethesda, MD), is constantly updated with information about genetic diseases. Another comprehensive compendium is *The Metabolic and Molecular Basis of Inherited Disease* by Scriver C, Beaudet A, Sly L, and Valle D, which provides excellent descriptions of the clinical and molecular aspects of genetic diseases. For the most up-to-date information, the scientific literature can be accessed without charge using PubMed (http://www.ncbi.nlm.nih.gov/PubMed).

We hope you find this volume useful in your clinical practice.

Contents

1. Congenital anatomic defects

AchondroplasiaSarcoidosis	2
Atelosteogenesis type 2	5
Campomelic dysplasia	7
Simpson-Golabi-Behmel syndrome	9
Smith-Lemli-Opitz syndrome	11

2. Disorders of the airway

Aspirin-induced asthma	14
Asthma	16
Cystic fibrosis	20
Keutel syndrome	25
Mucopolysaccharidosis type I	27
Mucopolysaccharidosis type II	30
Primary ciliary dyskinesia syndrome	32
Pseudohypoaldosteronism type 1	34
Pycnodysostosis	36
X-linked chondrodysplasia punctata	38

3. Disorders of alveoli

Alpha$_1$-Antichymotrypsin deficiency	42
Alpha$_1$-Antitrypsin deficiency	44
Chronic obstructive pulmonary disease	48
Congenital alveolar proteinosis	51
Cutis laxa	53
Fabry's disease	55
Lysinuric protein intolerance	57
Neonatal respiratory distress syndrome	59

4. Infiltrative lung disorders

Farber's lipogranulomatosis **62**
Gaucher's disease **65**
Globoid cell leukodystrophy **69**
Niemann-Pick disease types A and B **71**
Niemann-Pick disease type C **74**

5. Interstitial lung disorders

Ankylosing spondylitis **78**
Dyskeratosis congenita **81**
Familial amyloidosis **83**
Familial interstitial lung disease **85**
Hermansky-Pudlak syndrome **87**

6. Disorders of the vasculature and blood

Hereditary hemorrhagic telangiectasia **90**
Familial primary pulmonary hypertension **92**
Sickle cell disease **94**

Disorders that predispose to pulmonary emboli:
Activated protein C resistance **97**
Antithrombin III deficiency **99**
Dysfibrinogenemia **101**
Hyperhomocysteinemia **103**
Protein C/protein S deficiencies **105**
Prothrombin gene mutation **107**

7. Disorders of the pleura/pleural space

Birt-Hogg-Dubé syndrome **110**
Ehlers-Danlos syndrome, vascular type **112**
Familial Mediterranean fever **114**
Marfan's syndrome **117**
TNF receptor-associated periodic syndromes **119**

8. Immunodeficiencies

Ataxia-telangiectasia 122
Bloom's syndrome 124
Chronic granulomatous disease 126
Hyper-IgE syndrome 128
Leukocyte mycobacterial defect 130
Major histocompatibility complex class I deficiency 132
Major histocompatibility complex class II deficiency 134
Severe combined immunodeficiency due to adenosine deaminase deficiency 136
Severe combined immunodeficiency, T-negative, B-positive 138
Severe combined immunodeficiency, T-negative, B-negative 140
Severe combined immunodeficiency due to Zap-70 deficiency 142
Wiskott-Aldrich syndrome 144
X-linked agammaglobulinemia 146
X-linked hyper-IgM syndrome 148

9. Neuromuscular diseases

Acid maltase deficiency 152
Amyotrophic lateral sclerosis 154
Congenital myasthenic syndromes 156
Muscular dystrophy, Duchenne and Becker types 158
Myotonic dystrophy 160
Myotubular myopathy 162
Nemaline myopathy 164
Spinal muscular atrophy 166

10. Other

Congenital central hypoventilation syndrome 170
Klinefelter's syndrome 173
Leigh disease 175
Lung cancer 177
Prader-Willi syndrome 179
Rett syndrome 181
Sarcoidosis 183
Tuberous sclerosis 186

11. Abbreviations 189

12. Glossary 193

13. Index 249

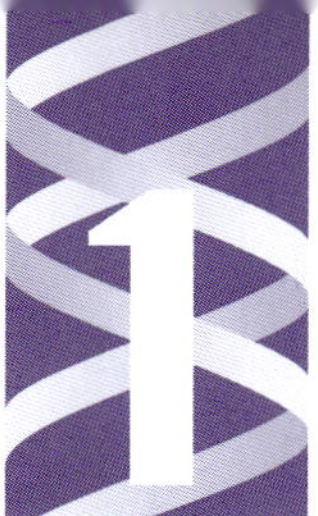

1. Congenital anatomic defects

Achondroplasia **2**

Atelosteogenesis type 2 **5**

Campomelic dysplasia **7**

Simpson-Golabi-Behmel syndrome **9**

Smith-Lemli-Opitz syndrome **11**

Achondroplasia

MIM 100800

Clinical features Respiratory problems, including obstructive and central sleep apnea, tachypnea, small airway damage, and hyperinflation – possibly secondary to gastroesophageal reflux disease and a small thoracic cavity – may progress to cor pulmonale, cardiorespiratory failure, and death. Other characteristics include short stature, rhizomelic short limbs, macrocephaly, midfacial hypoplasia, hydrocephalus, small foramen magnum, recurrent otitis media, lumbar lordosis, trident hand, tibial bowing, and obesity.

Age of onset Birth, but can be suspected during pregnancy.

Epidemiology 1:25 000

Inheritance Autosomal dominant, but most cases are not familial.

Chromosomal location 4p16.3

Genes The fibroblast growth factor receptor 3 gene (*FGFR3*) spans 19 exons extending over 16.5 kb.

Fibroblast growth factors are involved in mesenchymal and neural cell differentiation and growth during development, angiogenesis, and apoptosis.

Mutational spectrum Almost all patients have a $G^{380}R$ mutation, usually due to a replacement of guanine (G) by adenine (A) at nucleotide 1138, encoding a transmembrane region of the protein. It is thought that this might be one of the most common areas for mutation in the entire human genome.

Effect of mutation

The $G^{380}R$ mutation causes constitutive activation of FGFR3, which normally inhibits the formation of bone, resulting in failure of differentiation and replication of chondrocytes at the cartilage growth plate of long bones. While there is some evidence to suggest that this occurs through downregulation of integrin subunits and actin stress fibers, the exact mechanism has not been elucidated.

Diagnosis

The diagnosis is usually made clinically and radiologically, but polymerase chain reaction (PCR) amplication and restriction enzyme digestion can be used to identify the $G^{380}R$ mutation.

Counselling issues

Adenotonsillectomy should be considered for patients with obstructive sleep apnea, and ventriculoperitoneal shunt placement or cervicomedullary decompression surgery, if clinically indicated, can reduce central apneic spells. Antireflux therapy can also be instituted to prevent potential lung damage.

Prenatal diagnosis using amniocytes can detect fetal mutations, but some have argued that this test should only be completed to rule out fetal homozygosity. Prenatal diagnosis by ultrasound is difficult, but can be attempted in the third trimester.

Related conditions

There are several other diseases due to mutations in *FGFR3*. Achondroplasia lies on a continuum of disease, with hypochondroplasia (MIM 146000) and thanatophoric dysplasia (MIM 187600) representing disorders with lesser and greater severity, respectively. Replacement of alanine by glutamate at codon 391 ($A^{391}E$) causes Crouzon's disease with acanthosis nigricans (MIM 123500). Muenke coronal craniosynostosis (MIM 602849) is due to a replacement of proline by arginine at codon 250 ($P^{250}R$) in *FGFR3*. Some patients with a $L^{650}M$ missense mutation develop thanatophoric dysplasia, whereas others develop SADDAN dysplasia (severe achondroplasia with developmental delay and acanthosis nigricans).

References

Tasker RC, Dundas I, Laverty A, et al. Distinct patterns of respiratory difficulty in young children with achondroplasia: a clinical, sleep, and lung function study. Arch Dis Child 1998;79:99–108.

Vajo Z, Francomano CA, Wilkin DJ. The molecular and genetic basis of fibroblast growth factor receptor 3 disorders: the achondroplasia family of skeletal dysplasias, Muenke craniosynostosis, and Crouzon syndrome with acanthosis nigricans. Endocr Rev 2000;21:23–39.

Atelosteogenesis Type 2

(also known as: Neonatal osseous dysplasia I; de la Chapelle dysplasia; AO II)

MIM	256050
Clinical features	Pulmonary hypoplasia and tracheobronchomalacia, due to scoliosis, kyphosis, and a narrow, bell-shaped chest, usually cause death within hours of birth. Abnormal cartilage and bone development results in markedly short limbs, prenatal growth retardation, cleft palate, abnormal facies, laryngeal stenosis, "hitch-hiker thumb", talipes equinovarus, and enlarged space between the first and second toes.
Age of onset	Birth
Epidemiology	The incidence is very low, but more common in Finland.
Inheritance	Autosomal recessive
Chromosomal location	5q32–q33.1
Genes	*DTDST*, encoding the 82-kD diastrophic dysplasia sulfate transporter, spans 8.4 kb and has four exons. The protein functions as a sodium-independent sulfate transporter in chondrocytes and aids in sulfation of proteoglycans in cartilage.
Mutational spectrum	A missense mutation in codon 279, causing a replacement of arginine with tryptophan, has been found in a significant proportion of subjects. Missense and frameshift mutations at other locations also cause disease.
Effect of mutation	The $R^{279}W$ mutation causes variable loss of function of the sulfate transporter, with resultant undersulfation of proteoglycans in the cartilage matrix, and abnormal cartilage and bone development. The abnormal bony thoracic cavity causes pulmonary hypoplasia and neonatal respiratory insufficiency.

Diagnosis

Diagnosis is based on distinctive radiologic characteristics and genomic DNA analysis of skin fibroblasts.

Counselling issues

Prenatal diagnosis can be established by fetal ultrasound and genomic DNA analysis of amniocytes.

Related conditions

AO II is on a continuum of diseases due to mutations in *DTDST*, which also includes diastrophic dysplasia (MIM 222600) and achondrogenesis type IB (MIM 600972).

The most common mutation in *DTDST*, the "Finnish mutation", a thymine (T) to cytosine (C) transition in a splice donor site of an untranslated exon, rarely causes AO II. The mutation is seen more frequently in diastrophic dystrophy.

References

Newbury-Ecob, R. Atelosteogenesis type 2. J Med Genet 1998; 35(1):49–53.

Rossi A, van der Harten HJ, Beemer FA, et al. Phenotypic and genotypic overlap between atelosteogenesis type 2 and diastrophic dysplasia. Hum Genet 1996; 98:657–661.

Campomelic Dysplasia

(also known as: CMD1)

MIM	114290
Clinical features	Respiratory distress, due to tracheomalacia, small thorax, micrognathia, hypotonia, and cleft palate, is the usual cause of death. Facial anomalies include macrocephaly, flat nasal bridge, and low set ears. Patients often present as karyotypical males with female or ambiguous genitalia, absence of the olfactory tract or bulb, congenital heart disease, and renal abnormalities. Radiologic findings include eleven pairs of ribs, talipes equinovarus, congenital dislocation of the hips, bowed tibiae, pretibial skin dimples, hypoplastic scapulae, and short first metacarpals.
Age of onset	Birth
Epidemiology	0.05–1.6:10 000
Inheritance	Autosomal dominant
Chromosomal location	17q24.3–q25.1
Genes	*SOX9*, encoding a 509-amino acid member of the SRY family of transcription factors, is involved in bone formation and testis development. It contains a high-mobility group domain, a region of unknown function with repeating proline, glutamine, and alanine residues, and a carboxy-terminal transactivation domain.
Mutational spectrum	Missense, nonsense, frameshift, and splice site mutations have been reported.
Effect of mutation	The phenotype appears to be a result of haploinsufficiency, where one normal allele is unable to compensate for the mutant allele. *SOX9* regulates the expression of type II collagen, the major matrix

protein of cartilage. Dysfunctional expression of type II collagen during chondrogenesis results in abnormal cartilage development in the trachea and skeleton. *SOX9* is also involved in Sertoli cell differentiation, which might explain the abnormality in male sex organ development.

Diagnosis

Diagnosis is based on single strand conformational polymorphism (SSCP) analysis of the *SOX9* gene, but can also be based on the radiological demonstration of hypoplastic scapulae, bowed femoral and/or tibial bones, vertically narrow iliac wings, and non-mineralized thoracic pedicles.

Counselling issues

Most patients die within the first 24 hours of life, although occasionally some survive through infancy. Prenatal diagnosis can be made by ultrasound. It is likely that these autosomal dominant mutations arise *de novo*.

References

Mansour S, Hall CM, Pembrey ME, et al. A clinical and genetic study of campomelic dysplasia. J Med Genet 1995;32:415–20.

Meyer J, Sudbeck P, Held M, et al. Mutational analysis of the SOX9 gene in campomelic dysplasia and autosomal sex reversal: lack of genotype/phenotype correlations. Hum Mol Genet 1997;6:91–8.

Simpson-Golabi-Behmel Syndrome

(also known as: Golabi-Rosen syndrome; Simpson dysmorphia syndrome; SGBS)

MIM 312870

Clinical features Pulmonary hypoplasia due to a congenital diaphragmatic defect may cause respiratory distress at birth. Patients may also have abnormal lung lobation. Other frequent findings include macrosomia and macrocephaly, "coarse" face, supernumerary nipples, pectus excavatum, polydactyly, inguinal/umbilical hernias, congenital heart defects, cardiac arrhythmias, organomegaly, dysplastic kidneys, muscular hypotonia, and increased risk of neoplasia.

Age of onset Birth

Epidemiology Rare

Inheritance The disease is X-linked recessive, but penetrance is variable in female carriers.

Chromosomal location Xq26

Genes *GPC3* is an eight-exon, 500-kb gene that encodes glypican-3, a cell-surface protein of the heparan sulfate proteoglycan family that is involved in cell signaling during morphogenesis.

Mutational spectrum Most of the mutations are large deletions that involve more than one exon, often near the centromeric end of the gene. One missense and several nonsense mutations also produce hardly any protein product. Some patients may have balanced translocations between the X chromosome and an autosomal chromosome.

Effect of mutation It has been postulated that members of the glypican family serve as coreceptors that help bring growth factor ligands near their cell-surface receptors. Other hypotheses are that glypicans induce conformational changes in the ligand-receptor complex, or that glypicans bind both ligand and receptor to enhance reaction rate. Regardless of the mechanism, all mutations, except the missense mutation, result in truncated proteins with abnormal tertiary structure.

Diagnosis

Diagnosis is suggested on clinical grounds, but can be confirmed by SSCP analysis of each exon followed by direct sequence analysis of the abnormally migrating band.

Counselling issues

Mortality is high in the neonatal period, often due to the abnormal development of the lungs or heart. Some patients, however, may live well into adulthood.

Related conditions

A second locus (MIM 300209) at chromosome Xp22 has been linked to a more severe form of the disease, but the gene is unknown.

References

Neri G, Gurrieri F, Zanni G, et al. Clinical and molecular aspects of the Simpson-Golabi-Behmel syndrome. Am J Med Genet 1998;79:279–83.

Selleck SB. Overgrowth syndromes and the regulation of signaling complexes by proteoglycans. Am J Hum Genet 1999;64:372–7.

Smith-Lemli-Opitz Syndrome

Type 1

(also known as: SLO syndrome Type 1; RSH syndrome)

Type 2

(also known as: Rutledge Lethal Multiple Congenital Anomaly Syndrome; SLO Syndrome Type 2; Lethal Acrodysgenital Syndrome)

MIM 270400 Type 1; 268670 Type 2

Clinical features Patients present with multiple congenital anomalies including pulmonary hypoplasia, abnormal lung lobation, and abnormalities of laryngeal and tracheal cartilage causing obstructive sleep apnea. Other characteristics include mental retardation, postnatal growth stunting, microcephaly, structural brain anomalies, facial abnormalities, cleft palate, congenital heart defects, pyloric stenosis, renal anomalies, ambiguous external genitalia in males, cryptorchidism, polydactyly, and "Y-shaped" second and third toe syndactyly. Type 2 disease is more severe than type 1.

Age of onset Birth

Epidemiology 1:20 000–40 000

Inheritance Autosomal recessive

Chromosomal location 11q12–q13

Genes The defect resides in *DHCR7*, a nine-exon gene that encodes the 54.5-kD 7-dehydrocholesterol reductase, the enzyme responsible for reducing the C7=C8 double bond of the sterol molecule in the last step of cholesterol biosynthesis.

Mutational spectrum Over 120 mutations have been identified. Most are missense mutations occurring near transmembrane domains, but over 1/4 of patients have a specific splice-site mutation in intron 8 (IVS8 – 1G→C).

Effect of mutation

The mutations are believed to impair normal interaction between cholesterol and the hedgehog family of proteins, which are critical in fetal development. The exact mechanism by which cholesterol or its precursors affect the hedgehog proteins or result in various deformities is unclear.

Diagnosis

Diagnosis is based on characteristic clinical findings, elevated serum 7-dehydrocholesterol (DHC) and 8-DHC, and mutational analysis of genomic DNA.

Counselling issues

Various feeding problems in infancy, including poor sucking and swallowing, often necessitate nasogastric or gastrostomy feeding tubes. While muscle tone is poor in the first year, it usually improves to normal in older children. Life expectancy is dependent on the severity of the anomalies and quality of the supportive care. Prenatal diagnosis can be suggested by low unconjugated estriol on maternal triple screen or an elevated level of 7-DHC in amniotic fluid.

SLO types 1 and 2 are part of a continuous spectrum of disease. The distinction was originally made because those with type 2 died during infancy, but some now claim that there should be no distinction between the two types.

References

Kelley RI, Hennekam RCM. The Smith-Lemli-Opitz syndrome. J Med Genet 2000; 37:321–35.

Waterham HR, Wijburg FA, Hennekam RC, et al. Smith-Lemli-Opitz syndrome is caused by mutations in the 7-dehydrocholesterol reductase gene. Am J Hum Genet 1998;63:329–38.

Yu H, Lee M-H, Starck L, et al. Spectrum of delta 7-dehydrocholesterol reductase mutations in patients with the Smith-Lemli-Opitz (RSH) syndrome. Hum Molec Genet 2000;9:1385–91.

2. Disorders of the airway

Aspirin-induced asthma **14**

Asthma **16**

Cystic fibrosis **20**

Keutel syndrome **25**

Mucopolysaccharidosis type I **27**

Mucopolysaccharidosis type II **30**

Primary ciliary dyskinesia syndrome **32**

Pseudohypoaldosteronism type I **34**

Pycnodysostosis **36**

X-linked chondrodysplasia punctata **38**

Aspirin-induced Asthma

(also known as: Aspirin intolerant asthma; Asthma, nasal polyps, and aspirin intolerance; Aspirin triad; AIA)

MIM 208550

Clinical features Rhinitis is the first symptom, usually precipitated by an upper respiratory viral infection. Within several months, nasal polyps are seen on examination and patients may report anosmia, rhinorrhea and/or nasal congestion, and intermittent or chronic sinusitis. Patients also develop sensitivity to aspirin. Within a few hours of ingesting aspirin or any other nonsteroidal anti-inflammatory drug (NSAID), an asthmatic attack ensues, similar to an immediate hypersensitivity response, consisting of extensive airway inflammation, severe wheezing, laryngospasm, rhinorrhea, periorbital edema, injection of the conjunctiva, and peripheral vasodilation of the head and neck. Many patients develop severe acute asthmatic attacks requiring mechanical ventilation.

Age of onset Early adulthood

Epidemiology Ten to twenty percent of asthmatic adults have aspirin-induced asthma (AIA), but the prevalence is greater in women than men.

Inheritance Multifactorial

Chromosomal location 5q35

Genes *LTC4S*, a 5-exon gene extending over 2.52 kb, encodes the 18-kD, 150-amino acid leukotriene C_4 (LTC_4) synthase, an enzyme that catalyzes the conversion of LTA_4 to LTC_4 in the 5-lipoxygenase pathway in mast cells, eosinophils, basophils, and macrophages. LTC_4, a member of the cysteinyl leukotriene family, is a proinflammatory factor that is an eosinophil attractant and constrictor of smooth muscle.

Mutational spectrum

About 25% of the general population, but up to 40% of those with AIA, have an adenine (A) to cytosine (C) transversion 444 nucleotides upstream from the translation start codon in the promoter region.

Effect of mutation

Aspirin and other NSAIDs inhibit cyclooxygenase activity, thereby decreasing synthesis of prostaglandin E_2 (PGE2). Since PGE2 inhibits the production of LTC_4, ingestion of an NSAID results in loss of inhibition of LTC_4 synthesis. In normal individuals this is not clinically important. In those with the variant polymorphism, however, increased transcription of LTC_4 synthase results in overproduction of LTC_4 and the AIA phenotype.

Diagnosis

The most common method of diagnosis is the oral aspirin challenge test. Patients are given increasing doses of aspirin in a controlled clinical setting. A greater than 20% decrease in forced expiratory volume in 1 second (FEV_1), along with rhinorrhea and ocular congestion, constitutes a "classic diagnosis". Those with lesser decreases in FEV_1 are diagnosed as having "partial asthma".

Counselling issues

Patients remain sensitive to NSAIDs throughout life. Presumably, additional genetic or environmental factors contribute to the etiology of the disease. Treatment for AIA is the same as for non-aspirin induced asthma. If an analgesic is required, patients may be able to take low doses of acetaminophen.

References

Bigby TD. The leukotriene C4 synthase gene and asthma. Am J Respir Cell Mol Biol 2000;23:273–276.

Szczeklik A, Stevenson DD. Aspirin-induced asthma: advances in pathogenesis and management. J Allergy Clin Immunol 1999;104:5–13.

Asthma

MIM

600807

Clinical features

Patients exhibit reversible airway obstruction with airway inflammation and hyperresponsiveness to various stimuli. Dyspnea, cough, and wheezing are classic complaints. During attacks of severe obstruction, patients may display pulsus paradoxus, nasal flaring, and use of accessory respiratory muscles, but absent wheezing. There is an association with atopic dermatitis and allergic rhinitis. Peak expiratory flow rates are decreased, and pulmonary function testing reveals an obstructive pattern. Provocation with agents such as methacholine may be useful in eliciting hyperresponsiveness, especially in patients with normal baseline pulmonary function tests.

Age of onset

Often appears first in childhood.

Epidemiology

About 15 million people in the United States are affected, 3–5 million of whom are children. It is the most common chronic disease of childhood, more frequent in cities than rural areas, and more prevalent in boys than girls, but sex differences disappear after puberty. African-Americans and Native-Americans are more severely affected, as are those in lower socioeconomic classes. Prevalence rates vary significantly among countries.

Inheritance

Asthma does not have a Mendelian inheritance pattern. It is clear from family studies that there is some genetic component involving multiple genes, and it appears that various combinations of polymorphisms in genes can produce disease in different families. Environmental influences also prominently affect prevalence.

Genes

The region 5q31–33 encodes a cluster of cytokines including IL-3, IL-4, IL-5, IL-9, the β-chain of IL-12, and IL-13 and also the β-adrenergic receptor, corticosteroid receptor, and granulocyte-macrophage colony-stimulating factor. Many studies have shown linkage to this region and polymorphisms in several genes have been associated with asthma, as shown in Table 1. Some of the cytokines (e.g. IL-4, IL-13) increase B cell Ig class switching to IgE by T_H2 helper T cells. Data must be interpreted with caution as some polymorphisms may be merely in linkage disequilibrium with neighboring genes instead of themselves affecting disease. Other loci on chromosomes 12q14–q24.2 and 14q11.2–q13 have been associated, but no genes have been identified.

Diagnosis

In the proper clinical setting, peak expiratory flow rate or spirometry may be used for diagnosis. In a setting where the diagnosis is less certain, repeated peak expiratory flow rates over time or provocative testing with an agent such as methacholine can be confirmatory.

References

Barnes KC. Atopy and asthma genes – where do we stand? Allergy 2000;55:803–17.

Los H, Koppelman GH, Postma DS. The importance of genetic influences in asthma. Eur Respir J 1999;14:1210–27.

Sandford AJ, Pare PD. The genetics of asthma. The important questions. Am J Respir Crit Care Med 2000;161:S202–6.

Gene	Locus	Polymorphism	Genetic Evidence	Functional significance
β_2-adrenergic receptor	5q32–q34	$Q^{27}E$	Case-control studies show lower prevalence and bronchial hyperreactivity	Desensitization by repeated receptor stimulation varies with the polymorphism
		$R^{16}G$	Greater prevalence of severe asthma and nocturnal asthma, and quicker tachyphylaxis to bronchodilators	
IL-4	5q31.1	-590C/T	Case-control studies demonstrate greater prevalence of asthma, atopic dermatitis, and elevated IgE levels	The polymorphism is in a transcription regulatory region that may affect serum IgE levels
β chain of the high-affinity IgE receptor	11q13	$E^{237}G$	Greater risk of asthma, atopy, and bronchial hyperresponsiveness	There is greater binding of IgE with resultant increased IL-4 expression
IL-4 receptor α	16p12.1–p11.2	$I^{50}V$	This polymorphism is associated with increased risk of asthma and atopy	Greater B cell growth and IgE expression in response to IL-4
IL-13	5q31	T allele at –1111 in 5´ promoter	Greater risk of asthma, bronchial hyperreactivity, and skin test sensitivity	These various polymorphisms enhance the ability of IL-13 to increase B cell expression of IgE
		A allele at 4738 in 3´ untranslated region	Greater risk of asthma and skin test sensitivity	
		$Q^{110}R$	Greater risk of asthma	

Gene	Locus	Polymorphism	Genetic Evidence	Functional significance
Glutathione S-transferase pi	11q13	Val^{105}/Val^{105}	Greater risk of asthma, bronchial hyperreactivity, and skin test sensitivity	Glutathione S-transferases regulate levels of reactive oxygen species (ROS). This polymorphism affects the enzyme's ability to detoxify ROS, which may lead to greater bronchial hyperreactivity and asthma
CD14	5q31.1	-159C/T	Lower levels of serum IgE	This polymorphism results in an increased shift from T helper (T_H)1 to T_H2 cells
Clara cell-specific 16 kD protein (CC16)	11q13	$A^{38}G$	Lower prevalence of asthma	This polymorphism affects the intensity of CC16 anti-inflammatory actions in the airway
TNF-α	6p21.3	-308G/A	Greater prevalence of asthma	This polymorphism in the promoter region might influence TNF-α expression, with effects on inflammation and bronchial hyperresponsiveness
IL-9	5q31.1	No polymorphism has been identified	This locus has been associated with increased bronchial hyperresponsiveness	IL-9 effects on T cell growth and development may increase numbers of T_H2 cells, promote mast cell growth, and cause release of IgE from primed B cells

Table 1. Partial list of polymorphisms that have been associated with disease prevalence in asthma.

Cystic Fibrosis

(also known as: CF)

MIM 219700

Clinical features

The clinical manifestations of disease are numerous, affecting primarily the lungs, pancreas, gastrointestinal tract, sweat glands, and reproductive system.

Deterioration of lung function due to the destructive effects of bacteria is the major determinant of morbidity and mortality. In early life, infants are colonized with *Staphylococcus aureus* and *Haemophilus influenzae*, but after the age of 2 most infections are due to *Pseudomonas aeruginosa*. Later in life, infection with *Burkholderia cepacia* may bring about rapid lung deterioration. Acute exacerbations of respiratory symptoms due to bacterial infections require hospitalization and intravenous antibiotics. Recurrent, severe inflammation, primarily due to neutrophils, causes bronchiectasis and extensive lung destruction. Airway hyperreactivity may become prominent. Mucus plugs are often seen at bronchoscopy and may contribute to atelectasis. Pneumothorax, due to ruptured apical blebs, occurs in a small percentage of patients. Nasal polyposis may be present. Allergic bronchopulmonary aspergillosis may aggravate wheezing or appear as new infiltrates on chest radiography. Other radiographic findings of the chest include peribronchial cuffing, flattened diaphragms, densities, opacities, and infiltrates. High-resolution computed tomography (CT) scanning reveals more details of lung pathology. Early changes in pulmonary function reflect small airway abnormalities (forced expiratory flow [FEF] 25–75%), but later FEV_1 becomes the most important predictor of lung function. When FEV_1 falls below 30% of predicted, the chance of mortality in the next 2 years is 50%. Patients should be placed on a transplant list at this time. Respiratory failure is the most common cause of death.

Over 80% of patients develop pancreatic insufficiency, characterized by the inability to secrete the fluid and enzymes necessary for digestion and absorption of fat and the fat-soluble vitamins A, D, E, and K. Failure to thrive due to the decreased absorption of fat and protein may be a presenting sign in childhood. Pancreatic enzyme replacement is necessary to correct the deficiency. Pancreatic fibrosis with fatty deposition distorts the normal architecture and causes death of the insulin-producing beta cells, leading to insulin-requiring diabetes mellitus. Patients who are pancreatic sufficient have an increased risk of developing acute and chronic pancreatitis.

About 20% of neonates with CF present at birth with meconium ileus that can be diagnosed and occasionally treated with a barium enema, although surgery, either with or without the removal of an intestinal segment, is often necessary. Later in life patients may develop distal intestinal obstruction syndrome due to a mechanism similar to meconium ileus. Rectal prolapse also occurs in a significant number of patients around the time of toilet training.

As life expectancy has increased, there has been an elevated incidence of hepatic and gall bladder disease, including fatty infiltration of the liver, biliary cirrhosis, and cholelithiasis.

Concentrations of chloride, sodium, and potassium in sweat are increased, leading parents to say that their child tastes salty. In very hot weather, patients can develop serum electrolyte abnormalities (hypochloremic metabolic alkalosis) requiring hospitalization.

Males are azoospermic due to congenital bilateral absence of the vas deferens while females may have decreased fertility.

Age of onset

Meconium ileus presents at birth. Patients are otherwise diagnosed on average by 4 years of age.

Epidemiology

About 1:3400 are affected with the disease and 1:25 are carriers. CF is the most common fatal autosomal recessive disorder and is more prevalent in whites.

Inheritance

Autosomal recessive

Chromosomal location 7q31.2

Genes The gene was cloned in 1989 and named *CFTR*, the cystic fibrosis transmembrane conductance regulator. The 27-exon gene, spread over 250 kb, encodes a 1480-amino acid protein with a predicted molecular mass of 168 kD. CFTR, a member of the adenosine triphosphate (ATP)-binding cassette family, is an ATP-dependent chloride channel on the apical surface of the cell with two nucleotide-binding and two membrane-spanning domains. In addition to its channel activity, CFTR regulates the function of other membrane proteins. In airway epithelial cells, CFTR inhibits the activity of the epithelial sodium channel (ENaC), but activates it in the sweat gland duct. CFTR affects the ability of cyclic adenosine monophosphate (cAMP) and cAMP-dependent protein kinase to activate the outward rectifying chloride channel. CFTR also regulates the function of a Cl^-/HCO_3^- exchanger in various cell types and a potassium channel in the renal collecting ducts.

Mutational spectrum Approximately 1000 mutations have been identified in the *CFTR* gene. The △F508 mutation comprises about $^2/_3$ of all mutant alleles. The missense mutations $G^{551}D$ and $N^{1303}K$, nonsense mutations $G^{542}X$ and $W^{1282}X$, and splice site mutations 621+1 G→T and 1717-1 G→T collectively make up about 8% of the mutant alleles worldwide. Almost half of all mutations are missense, whereas $^1/_4$ are frameshift insertions and deletions. Certain mutations occur more frequently in specific populations, such as $G^{551}D$ in Celts and $Y^{112}X$ in those from Reunion Island.

Effect of mutation There are four classes of mutation based on the mechanisms that cause dysfunction. Class I mutations, usually nonsense, frameshift, or splicing, cause reduced levels of protein, often because of messenger ribonucleic acid (mRNA) instability. Class II mutations, such as △F508, result from in-frame deletions, insertions, or missense mutations, causing dysfunctional folding, improper processing, and degradation of the protein. Class III mutations, most often due to missense mutations in nucleotide-binding domains

(NBDs), result from altered regulation of the open probability of the channel, usually due to abnormal interactions of ATP with an NBD. Lastly, class IV mutations are often due to missense mutations in the membrane-spanning domains, which affect the ability of ions to traverse the channel.

Exactly how mutations in *CFTR* cause lung disease has not been elucidated. The current theory focuses on abnormalities in salt-sensitive components of the innate immune system within airway surface liquid (ASL). High concentrations of sodium chloride within the ASL inhibit the antimicrobial action of enzymes such as β-defensins 1 and 2, lysozyme, and lactoferrin, allowing infection and colonization by microbes, and possibly causing a compensatory increase in inflammatory cells (e.g. neutrophils) and other components of the immune system. There is another theory that mutations in *CFTR* cause dysregulation of ENaCs with increased reabsorption of salt and fluid from the ASL. The reduced volume of ASL decreases mucociliary clearance and permits bacterial colonization.

Diagnosis

Diagnosis should be based on the characteristic manifestations (pulmonary, gastrointestinal, nutritional, electrolyte, and urogenital abnormalities), history of CF in a sibling, or a positive neonate screening test (e.g. immunoreactive trypsinogen). An elevated pilocarpine iontophoresis sweat test, demonstration of mutations in the *CFTR* gene, or abnormal *in vivo* nasal mucosa potential difference measurements is confirmatory.

Counselling issues

Median survival is 32 years, but males tend to live about 2 years longer than females. Genotype-phenotype relationships are clear, as certain mutations are associated with severe lung disease, meconium ileus, pancreatic status, and fertility. Polymorphisms in other genes besides *CFTR*, such as mannose-binding lectin, may influence the course of pulmonary disease. Second-hand cigarette smoke has been implicated in disease severity. Parents should be cautious about placing a child with CF in day care because of the high risk of viral infections, which can precipitate exacerbations. All patients more than 6 months of age should receive influenza vaccination annually. Pregnant women with CF are susceptible to worse lung disease, malnutrition, and an increased risk of gestational diabetes.

Related conditions

Some mutations in *CFTR* are associated with isolated congenital bilateral absence of the vas deferens (277180).

References

Davidson DJ, Porteous DJ. The genetics of cystic fibrosis lung disease. Thorax 1998;53:389–97.

Rosenstein BJ, Cutting GR. The diagnosis of cystic fibrosis: a consensus statement. J Pediatr 1998;132:589–94.

Welsh MJ, Ramsey BW, Accurso F, Cutting GR. Cystic fibrosis. In: Scriver CR, Beaudet AL, Sly WS, Valle D, editors. The Metabolic and Molecular Basis of Inherited Disease. 8th ed. New York: McGraw-Hill; 2001. p. 5121–88.

Wine JJ. The genesis of cystic fibrosis lung disease. J Clin Invest 1999;103:309–12.

Keutel Syndrome

MIM

245150

Clinical features

Upper and lower respiratory infections and wheezing are characteristic. An almost universal finding is premature calcification of cartilage in the larynx, trachea, nose, auricles, epiglottis, and costochondral joints. Peripheral pulmonary vascular stenoses may lead to pulmonary hypertension and right ventricular hypertrophy. Other characteristics include brachytelephalangism, characteristic facies including midface hypoplasia, mixed or conductive hearing defects, ventricular septal defect, and mild mental retardation.

Age of onset

Childhood to adolescence

Epidemiology

The disease is very rare with fewer than 20 cases reported.

Inheritance

Autosomal recessive

Chromosomal location

12p13.1–p12.3

Genes

The matrix Gla protein (*MGP*) gene has four exons, covers 3.9 kb, and encodes an 84-amino acid protein with a γ-carboxyglutamic acid-containing domain. This vitamin K-dependent protein is thought to be involved in extracellular matrix and bone calcification.

Mutational spectrum

Three mutations have been identified: a one base-pair deletion in exon 1 (c.69delG), a splice-acceptor site mutation (IVS1-2 A→G), and a nonsense mutation in exon 1 (c.113T→A).

Effect of mutation

Different mutations result in either truncated or absent proteins. Because of morphologic similarities to other disorders of calcification, it is thought that the defect is in a common vitamin K-dependent pathway that disrupts cartilage and skeletal development.

Diagnosis

Diagnosis can be made based on the constellation of findings, including abnormal calcification, brachytelephalanges, abnormal facies, and peripheral pulmonary stenoses. With the recent identification of the causative gene, direct sequence analysis of genomic DNA can confirm the diagnosis.

Counselling issues

Patients have a slight developmental delay, but normal life expectancy.

Related conditions

Because of the shared finding of midface hypoplasia, Binder syndrome (MIM 155050) may be a variant of Keutel syndrome.

References

Munroe PB, Olgunturk RO, Fryns JP, et al. Mutations in the gene encoding the human matrix Gla protein cause Keutel syndrome. Nature Genet 1999;21:142–4.

Teebi AS, Lambert DM, Kaye GM, et al. Keutel syndrome: further characterization and review. Am J Med Genet 1998;78:182–7.

Mucopolysaccharidosis Type I

(also known as: Hurler's syndrome; Hurler-Scheie syndrome; Scheie's syndrome)

MIM 258200

Clinical features

Type IH (Hurler's syndrome)

The upper airway becomes significantly obstructed by accumulation of glycosaminoglycans in the trachea and oropharynx, usually first noted as sleep apnea but progressing to daytime hypoxemia. Adenotonsillectomy may reduce symptomatology, but does not affect narrowing of the distal airway. Nasal continuous positive airway pressure (CPAP) and tracheostomy may also provide some relief. Macroglossia, small pharynx, small nasal airway, and short neck, in addition to the risk of spinal cord compression during hyperextension, make airway intubation very difficult. Skeletal abnormalities affecting the bony thorax cause restrictive ventilatory defects. Chronic rhinitis and upper respiratory infections are common, and pneumonia may be the cause of death. Other abnormalities include hydrocephalus, distinctive facies, corneal clouding, glaucoma, deafness, lumbar kyphoscoliosis, hepatosplenomegaly, and regression of neurodevelopmental skills.

Type IH/S (Hurler-Scheie syndrome)

The phenotype, including upper airway obstruction, is less severe than that of Type IH.

Type IS (Scheie's syndrome)

These patients are the most mildly affected, with infrequent upper airway obstruction and sleep apnea. Visual impairment due to corneal clouding is often the first symptom. There are usually minimal or no intellectual deficiencies.

Age of onset

Hurler's syndrome presents by the age of 2 years, Hurler-Scheie syndrome between 3 and 8 years, and Scheie's syndrome in the second decade.

Epidemiology 1:100 000–150 000

Inheritance Autosomal recessive

Chromosomal location 4p16.3

Genes The 19-kb, 14-exon *IDUA* gene encodes the 70-kD α-L-iduronidase, which cleaves terminal α-L-iduronic acid residues in the degradation of heparan sulfate and dermatan sulfate.

Mutational spectrum More than 50 mutations have been identified, most of which are missense or nonsense. The $W^{402}X$ and $Q^{70}X$ premature terminations are the predominant mutations in most populations.

Effect of mutation In general, Hurler's syndrome is due to the presence of two alleles with minimal activity. Either the protein is improperly processed or transported within the endoplasmic reticulum, or there is greatly diminished catalytic activity, resulting in accumulation of mucopolysaccharides. Patients with Hurler-Scheie and Scheie's syndromes have at least one allele with adequate residual activity.

Diagnosis Depending on the ethnic origin of the patient, PCR and restriction fragment digestion can detect certain mutations. Direct sequence analysis can be performed if PCR is unsuccessful.

Counselling issues Almost all patients with Hurler syndrome die by the age of 10 years from pneumonia or cardiac complications. Those with Hurler-Scheie syndrome may live into the third decade, and those with Scheie syndrome have a near normal life expectancy. Recombinant α-L-iduronidase, recently available, ameliorates some clinical features of the disease.

References

Neufeld EF, Muenzer J. The mucopolysaccharidoses. In: Scriver CR, Beaudet AL, Sly WS, Valle D, editors. The Metabolic and Molecular Basis of Inherited Disease. 8th ed. New York: McGraw-Hill; 2001. p. 3421–52.

Scott HS, Bunge S, Gal A, et al. Molecular genetics of mucopolysaccharidosis Type I: diagnostic, clinical, and biological implications. Hum Mutat 1995;6:288–302.

Mucopolysaccharidosis Type II

(also known as: Hunter's syndrome; Iduronate 2-sulfatase deficiency)

MIM	309900
Clinical features	Accumulation of mucopolysaccharide in the trachea and oropharynx, macroglossia, pharyngeal hypertrophy, adenoid hypertrophy, and excessive rhinorrhea cause upper airway obstruction, sleep apnea, and daytime hypoxemia. Distortion of cartilage in the airway begins proximally but eventually progresses to the distal airways. Cardiac valve dysfunction and coronary artery thickening may be the principal causes of death. Prominent characteristics include stiff joints, short stature, ivory-colored skin lesions on the back, abnormal facies, and hearing loss. A more severe form includes mental retardation, hydrocephalus, retinal degeneration, chronic diarrhea, and hepatomegaly.
Age of onset	The severe form presents by 3 years of age, whereas the mild form manifests in mid-childhood.
Epidemiology	1:100 000–200 000
Inheritance	X-linked recessive
Chromosomal location	Xq28
Genes	Iduronate-2-sulfatase, a 550-amino acid protein encoded in nine exons spread over the 24-kb *IDS* gene, is the enzyme responsible for removing sulfate from iduronic acid residues in the degradation of the mucopolysaccharides dermatan sulfate and heparan sulfate.
Mutational spectrum	Single amino acid changes causing missense and nonsense mutations are the most common, but small insertions and deletions represent a sizable minority of mutations. Mutations have been found to cluster in exons 3, 8, and 9.

Effect of mutation

Those patients with nonsense mutations, or large deletions, insertions, or rearrangements usually have severe disease, whereas those with missense mutations have a milder phenotype. Decreased sulfatase activity results in the accumulation of abnormal mucopolysaccharides.

Diagnosis

Diagnosis can be confirmed by SSCP analysis followed by genomic sequencing.

Counselling issues

Death usually occurs in the second decade in severe cases, but mild cases may live until the fifth or sixth decades.

Related conditions

Other types of mucopolysaccharidoses are due to defects in different enzymes in the heparan sulfate, keratan sulfate, chondroitin sulfate, and dermatan sulfate degradation pathways. In the various subsets of Type III, known as Sanfilippo syndrome (MIM 252900, 252920, 252930, 252940), asymptomatic patients may have increased interstitial markings on chest X-ray. In Type IV, Morquio syndrome (MIM 253000, 253010), skeletal deformities cause a restrictive ventilatory defect and upper airway obstruction, which may result in significant hypoxemia. Those with the neonatal form of Type VII, Sly syndrome (MIM 253220), develop hydrops fetalis and severe hypoventilation.

References

Li P, Bellows AB, Thompson JN. Molecular basis of iduronate-2-sulphatase gene mutations in patients with mucopolysaccharidosis type II (Hunter syndrome). J Med Genet 1999;36:21–7.

Neufeld EF, Muenzer J. The mucopolysaccharidoses. In: Scriver CR, Beaudet AL, Sly WS, Valle D, editors. The Metabolic and Molecular Basis of Inherited Disease. 8th ed. New York: McGraw-Hill; 2001. p. 3421–52.

Primary Ciliary Dyskinesia (PCD)

(also known as: Immotile ciliary syndrome [ICS]; Polynesian bronchiectasis)

MIM 242650

Clinical features Patients present with copious sputum production, lobar atelectasis, clubbing, wheezing, and radiographic evidence of bronchiectasis. Respiratory failure, pneumothorax, and hemoptysis are rare. An obstructive pattern on pulmonary function tests may be seen in older children. Other characteristics include sinusitis, male infertility due to immotile sperm, otitis media leading to conductive hearing loss, and nasal polyps.

Age of onset Depending on disease severity, presentation may be in childhood or later.

Epidemiology 1:20 000

Inheritance Autosomal recessive

Chromosomal location 9p21–p13

Genes The only known mutations have been found in *DNAI1*, dynein axonemal intermediate chain 1, a 699-amino acid, 78-kD, component of dynein. Axonemal dyneins move microtubule segments within cilia and flagella using an adenosine triphosphatase (ATPase)-dependent mechanism. Dynein is composed of inner and outer arms. The outer arm contains two heavy chains, two or more intermediate chains, and between four and eight light chains. The inner arm has a slightly more complicated structure and plays a greater role in waveform movement of cilia and flagella.

Mutational spectrum Known mutations in *DNAI1* are a 1-bp insertion (T) at nucleotide +3 of the intronic splice donor sequence following exon 1 and a 4-bp insertion (AATA) at codon 95.

Effect of mutation

Cilia within the respiratory tract create a flow of mucus towards the mouth, eliminating unwanted elements from the bronchial tree. A defect in any of the microtubule components could cause abnormal waveform motion altered beat frequency, or immotile cilia that result in ineffective mucociliary clearance, leading to retention of pathogens within the lung, chronic infection, and bronchiectasis. The mutations in *DNAI1* result in absence of the outer arms of dynein and loss of waveform movement of cilia.

Diagnosis

For patients older than 12 years, mucociliary clearance testing may be an appropriate first step, although rarely used. For younger patients, bronchoscopic ciliary brush scrapings of epithelial cells from the middle or inferior turbinate may be helpful in diagnosis, revealing abnormal ciliary waveforms on light microscopic examination. Many clinicians, however, rely on the clinical picture and electron microscopy of nasal cilia.

Counselling issues

Men are likely to be infertile, but there are reports of normal fertility. Absence of cilia in fallopian tubes may lead to a higher rate of ectopic pregnancy. Prevalence is high among New Zealand Maori and Samoan Islanders. Other genes besides *DNAI1* almost surely exist.

Related conditions

Kartagener's syndrome (MIM 244400) has the same manifestations but also includes situs inversus. The absence of dynein arms in cilia causes ineffective ciliary waveforms. Rotation of internal organs during development is believed to be dependent on the cilia of intestinal cells. When they are abnormal, rotation occurs randomly. The gene, thought to encode the dynein heavy chain, has been localized to 14qter.

References

Pennarun G, Escudier E, Chapelin C, et al. Loss-of-function mutations in a human gene related to Chlamydomonas reinhardtii dynein IC78 result in primary ciliary dyskinesia. Am J Hum Genet 1999;65:1508–19.

Meeks M, Bush A. Primary ciliary dyskinesia (PCD). Pediatr Pulmonol 2000;29:307–16.

Pseudohypoaldosteronism Type 1

(also known as: PHA1)

MIM 264350

Clinical features Patients develop recurrent bronchopneumonia from *Staphylococcus aureus*, *Pseudomonas aeruginosa,* and other organisms as in cystic fibrosis, but bronchiectasis does not occur. There is severe salt-wasting from the kidneys, colon, sweat ducts, and salivary glands. Metabolic abnormalities include hyperkalemia, hypovolemia, hyperaldosteronemia, metabolic acidosis, and hyperreninemia.

Age of onset Neonatal period

Epidemiology Rare

Inheritance Autosomal recessive

Chromosomal location *SCNN1A*; 12p13
SCNN1B and *SCNN1G*; 16p13–p12

Genes Defects have been found in *SCNN1A*, *SCNN1B*, and *SCNN1G*, encoding the α, β, and γ subunits of the amiloride-sensitive ENaC, respectively. ENaC, a heterotetramer of two α, one β, and one γ subunits, is located in the apical membrane of the cell and controls sodium reabsorption in the distal renal tubule, colon, sweat ducts, and salivary glands. The gene for the α subunit is on chromosome 12 while those for the β and γ subunits are in the same region of chromosome 16. The α subunit, the product of a 17-kb gene comprising 13 exons, has intrinsic channel activity, whereas the β (640 amino acids, 73 kD) and γ (649 amino acids, 74 kD) subunits serve as allosteric modifiers that significantly augment the activity of the α subunit.

Mutational spectrum

Eleven mutations have been identified in *SCNN1A*, ten resulting in truncated proteins and one causing an amino acid replacement. The only mutations in the other genes are a $G^{37}S$ replacement in *SCNN1B* and a 3-prime splice site mutation in intron A of *SCNN1G* (318–1 G→A).

Effect of mutation

Mutations affect the open probability of the channel, insertion of subunits into the membrane, or assembly and configuration of subunits, resulting in decreased channel conductance. Pulmonary symptoms are due to the increased volume of exudate within bronchioles, which reduces airway diameter and dilutes proteins that stabilize the airway surface.

Diagnosis

Diagnosis is based on severe salt wasting discovered in infancy with hyponatremia, hyperkalemia, metabolic acidosis, hyperreninemia, and hyperaldosteronemia. Mutational analysis of the three subunits from leukocytes or nasal epithelium is confirmatory.

Counselling issues

Salt replacement is required in the first few years of life but may be less critical after infancy. The severity of pulmonary disease usually decreases with age.

Related conditions

An autosomal dominant form of this disorder results from a mutation in the gene for the mineralocorticoid receptor (MIM 600983). Another condition, Liddle syndrome (MIM 177200), characterized by hypervolemia, hypokalemia, and metabolic alkalosis, is caused by inappropriate activation of the ENaC receptor due to mutations in the β or γ subunits.

References

Schaedel C, Marthinsen L, Kristoffersson AC, et al. Lung symptoms in pseudohypoaldosteronism type 1 are associated with deficiency of the alpha-subunit of the epithelial sodium channel. J Pediatr 1999;135:739–45.

Kerem E, Bistritzer T, Hanukoglu A, et al. Pulmonary epithelial sodium-channel dysfunction and excess airway liquid in pseudohypoaldosteronism. N Engl J Med 1999;341:156–62.

Pycnodysostosis

(also known as: Cathepsin K deficiency)

MIM	265800
Clinical features	Upper airway obstruction, due to a long soft palate, retrognathia with glossoptosis, and a low hanging uvula, causes obstructive sleep apnea, carbon dioxide retention, and, in some patients, may lead to pulmonary hypertension and right-sided heart failure. Skeletal abnormalities are prominent, including short stature, shortened phalanges, macrocephaly, osteosclerosis, and easy fracturing. Dental anomalies and growth hormone deficiency are often present.
Age of onset	Birth
Epidemiology	Rare
Inheritance	Autosomal recessive
Chromosomal location	1q21
Genes	The 11-kb *CTSK* gene comprises eight exons on chromosome 1, encoding the 30-kD cathepsin K, a cysteine protease expressed almost exclusively in osteoclasts that is necessary for bone resorption.
Mutational spectrum	Eleven of the twelve reported mutations are due to single base changes, resulting in amino acid replacement or premature termination. One single base deletion has also been reported.
Effect of mutation	Normally, osteoclasts degrade bone matrix, ingest collagen and other protein components by endocytosis, translocate the vesicles to the basolateral membrane, and secrete the content into the extracellular space. Ineffective proteolysis of collagen fibrils in those with cathepsin K mutations interferes with osteoclastic removal of the

organic matrix in bone, resulting in osteosclerosis and other skeletal anomalies.

Diagnosis

Diagnosis is made by the characteristic radiologic and clinical features.

Counselling issues

Diligent dental care is necessary to prevent and treat caries, and susceptibility to osteomyelitis of the jaw following tooth extractions must be recognized. Life span appears to be normal.

It is hypothesized that a carrier advantage accounts for persistence of the allele. Heterozygotes may be protected from osteoporosis without the pathologic abnormalities of pycnodysostosis.

Related conditions

The differential diagnosis includes osteopetrosis (MIM 259700), osteogenesis imperfecta (MIM 166200), sclerosteosis (MIM 269500), and endosteal hyperostosis (MIM 144750), but the usual radiologic appearance or inheritance pattern of each is different.

References

Aronson DC, Heymans HS, Bijlmer RP. Cor pulmonale and acute liver necrosis, due to upper airway obstruction as part of pycnodysostosis. Eur J Pediatr 1984;141:251–3.

Gelb BD, Bromme D, Desnick RJ. Pycnodysostosis: cathepsin K deficiency. In: Scriver CR, Beaudet AL, Sly WS, Valle D, editors. The Metabolic and Molecular Basis of Inherited Disease. 8th ed. New York: McGraw-Hill; 2001. p. 3453–68.

X-linked Chondrodysplasia Punctata

Type 1

(also known as: CPXR; CDPX1)

Type 2

(also known as: Conradi-Hünermann syndrome; Happle syndrome; Conradi-Hünermann-Happle syndrome; CPXD; CDPX2)

MIM 302950 Type 1; 302960 Type 2

Clinical features Abnormal calcium deposition in the larynx and trachea and choanal stenosis lead to respiratory distress soon after birth, but usually resolve by 3 years of age. Restrictive lung disease results from an abnormally shaped chest wall.

Type 1
Other characteristics in Type 1 include punctate calcifications on chest X-ray, nasal hypoplasia, short stature, hypoplastic distal phalanges, alopecia, patent ductus arteriosus, ventricular septal defect, deafness, and short neck.

Type 2
Features characteristic in Type 2 include punctate calcifications on chest X-ray, abnormal facies with flattened nasal bridge, joint contractures, scoliosis, kyphosis, linear ichthyosis and other keratotic and pigmentary abnormalities, cataracts, alopecia, and malformed nails.

Age of onset Neonatal to adolescence

Epidemiology Rare

Inheritance Type 1, X-linked recessive; Type 2, X-linked dominant

Chromosomal location *ARSE*; Xp22.3
EBP; Xp11.23–p11.22

Genes

Type 1

The *ARSE* gene, which encodes the 68-kD arylsulfatase E, is located in a region of the X chromosome that contains two other arylsulfatases. Arylsulfatase E, similar to all sulfatases, hydrolyzes sulfate ester bonds in various molecular compounds that are thought to be present in cartilage and bone matrix.

Type 2

EBP is a 5-exon, 1.0-kb gene that encodes the △8–△7-sterol isomerase, also known as emopamil binding protein, an enzyme that catalyzes the conversion of cholest-8(9)-en-3beta-ol to cholest-7-en-3beta-ol in cholesterol and vitamin D syntheses. The 25- to 27-kD protein contains 230 amino acids and has four predicted membrane-spanning domains.

Mutational spectrum

Type 1

Several missense mutations and one nonsense mutation are known.

Type 2

Many are null mutations, either nonsense or frameshift, encoding a truncated protein. Several missense and splice-site mutations also exist. Nucleotides 293 to 298 may represent a "hot spot" for mutations.

Effect of mutation

Type 1

Most mutations result in decreased catalytic activity of the enzyme, presumably through abnormal folding and tertiary structure.

Type 2

The phenotype may be due to the accumulation of toxic cholesterol pathway intermediates upstream from the substrate of the mutated enzyme, but the exact mechanism has not been elucidated.

Diagnosis

The diagnosis is based on characteristic punctate calcifications seen radiologically, and sequence analysis of genomic DNA can be confirmatory.

Counselling issues

Almost all cases of Type 2 have been in females. Although it was originally suggested that males die *in utero*, it is now postulated that males are selectively spared from the disease, but can transmit it to female children. Severity of disease in the female is related to lyonization of the X-chromosome. In the absence of restrictive lung disease, life expectancy is normal.

Related conditions

It is thought that warfarin embryopathy results from inadequate arylsulfatase E activity. Vitamin K epoxide reductase deficiency (MIM 277450) is also associated with punctate calcifications.

References

Daniele A, Parenti G, d'Addio M, et al. Biochemical characterization of arylsulfatase E and functional analysis of mutations found in patients with X-linked chondrodysplasia punctata. Am J Hum Genet 1998;62:562–72.

Franco B, Meroni G, Parenti G, et al. A cluster of sulfatase genes on Xp22.3: mutations in chondrodysplasia punctata (CDPX) and implications for warfarin embryopathy. Cell 1995;81:15–25.

Has C, Bruckner-Tuderman L, Muller D, et al. The Conradi-Hünermann-Happle syndrome (CDPX2) and emopamil binding protein: novel mutations, and somatic and gonadal mosaicism. Hum Mol Genet 2000;9:1951–5.

Kelley RI, Wilcox WG, Smith M, et al. Abnormal sterol metabolism in patients with Conradi-Hünermann-Happle syndrome and sporadic lethal chondrodysplasia punctata. Am J Med Genet 1999;83:213–19.

Seguin JH, Baugh RF, McIntee RA. Airway manifestations of chondrodysplasia punctata. Int J Pediatr Otorhinolaryngol 1993;27:85–90.

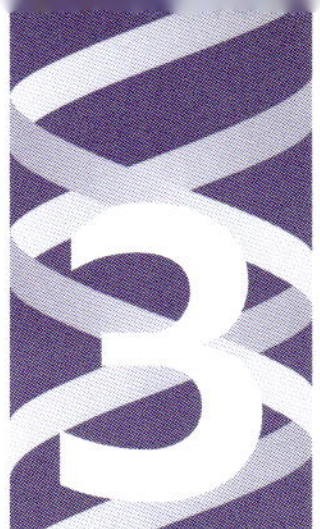

3. Disorders of alveoli

Alpha$_1$-Antichymotrypsin deficiency **42**

Alpha$_1$-Antitrypsin deficiency **44**

Chronic obstructive pulmonary disease **48**

Congenital alveolar proteinosis **51**

Cutis laxa **53**

Fabry's disease **55**

Lysinuric protein intolerance **57**

Neonatal respiratory distress syndrome **59**

Alpha$_1$-antichymotrypsin Deficiency

(also known as: AACT; ACT)

MIM 107280

Clinical features Patients present with chronic obstructive pulmonary disease (COPD) and an obstructive pattern in pulmonary function tests. Symptoms include cough, dyspnea, and wheezing. Childhood asthma and hepatic cirrhosis may also be associated.

Age of onset Adulthood

Epidemiology The gene frequency in Sweden is 0.3%; other populations have not been studied.

Inheritance Autosomal dominant

Chromosomal location 14q32.1

Genes *ACT* encodes α_1-antichymotrypsin, a 68-kD member of the serine protease inhibitor class of proteins. Alpha$_1$-antichymotrypsin inhibits cathepsin G and is an acute phase reactant whose serum levels increase in response to stress, infection, and trauma. It has a serum concentration approximately one-tenth that of α_1-antitrypsin.

Mutational spectrum The Bonn mutation at position 229, resulting in an alanine replacement by proline, and the Bochum mutation, replacement of proline by leucine at position 55, are the only mutations known to cause clinical disease.

Effect of mutation The mutations probably decrease α_1-antichymotrypsin secretion, resulting in persistent activation of cathepsin G, a neutrophil chemo-attractant and proteinase that may damage lung tissues.

Diagnosis

Diagnosis is based on plasma concentrations of α_1-antichymotrypsin, with confirmation by sequence analysis of genomic DNA.

Counselling issues

A replacement of alanine by threonine at codon 15 in α_1-antichymotrypsin, when present with a specific polymorphism of the *APOE4* gene, may confer an increased risk of Alzheimer's disease. In addition, there may be an increased risk of Parkinson's disease with the α_1-antichymotrypsin alanine to threonine polymorphism, independent of the *APOE4* allele.

References

Poller W, Faber JP, Weidinger S, et al. A leucine-to-proline substitution causes a defective α_1-antichymotrypsin allele associated with familial obstructive lung disease. Genomics 1993;17:740–43.

Alpha$_1$-antitrypsin deficiency

(also known as: Protease inhibitor 1 deficiency; Anti-elastase deficiency; AAT deficiency)

MIM

107400

Clinical features

Emphysema, usually in the lung bases, is one of the defining pathologies of the disease. Patients complain of dyspnea, wheezing, chronic cough productive of sputum, and hay fever. Forced expiratory volume in 1 second (FEV_1) is markedly reduced, but patients may be responsive to bronchodilators. Pathologic examination shows panacinar involvement with loss of elastic recoil and destruction of attachments that support small airways, which is the cause of irreversible airway obstruction. In addition, goblet cell metaplasia, smooth muscle hyperplasia, fibrosis, inflammatory cells, and luminal secretion in the bronchioles produce reversible airway obstruction. Cigarette smoking is a major risk factor for earlier onset and greater severity of disease. History of pneumonia and parental history of emphysema are also risk factors. Chronic bronchitis may also be present, and asthma and bronchiectasis are reported in a small percentage of patients.

Liver fibrosis is the other cardinal manifestation. Alpha$_1$-antitrypsin deficiency is one of the predominant reasons for liver transplantation in children. Pathologic examination of liver biopsies reveals α_1-antitrypsin in periportal hepatocytes. As the disease worsens, fibrosis, bile duct proliferation, hepatocyte metaplasia, and hepatocellular carcinoma may occur. The incidence of liver disease is higher in males.

Age of onset

Presentation varies with smoking history. COPD develops in about the fifth decade.

Epidemiology

PI ZZ occurs in 1:3000–6000 North Americans. Two to three percent of COPD cases in the US are due to α_1-antitrypsin deficiency.

Inheritance Autosomal recessive

Chromosomal location 14q32.1

Genes The *PI* gene encodes the protease inhibitor, α_1-antitrypsin. It contains seven exons spanning 12.2 kb, but only 1.4 kb in four exons encode the 52-kD protein product. Alpha$_1$-antitrypsin is a member of the serpin (serine protease inhibitor) family along with α_1-antichymotrypsin, protein C inhibitor, and cortisol-binding globulin. These proteins are encoded adjacent to PI on chromosome 14, and have substantial sequence similarity. Alpha$_1$-antitrypsin contains nine α helices and three β sheets. Exon 5 contains both the active site and the stop codon. The protein is primarily synthesized in the liver, but there is some production in monocytes and other cells. Hepatocytes and macrophages use different promoter regions, located in exons Ic and Ia, respectively.

Mutational spectrum About 100 alleles have been identified, the most common being functional PI M subtypes. The most prevalent mutant allele that produces disease is PI Z, a missense mutation at codon 342, causing replacement of glutamate with lysine in exon 5. The PI S allele, Glu^{264}Val, is another common mutation.

Effect of mutation Normal levels of α_1-antitrypsin in the serum range from 20–53 μmol/L, but it is thought that pathology is not commonly seen at levels above 11 μmol/L. Patients with PI ZZ and other severe mutations have levels of approximately 5–6 μmol/L as a result of normal synthesis, but impaired secretion of the mutant protein. In the tertiary structure of the normal protein molecule, the negatively charged glutamate at codon 342 is adjacent to the positively charged lysine at codon 290. The lysine variant at codon 342 in PI Z does not form the bridge required for normal protein folding.

A precise balance between proteases and antiproteases is necessary for normal lung function. Neutrophil elastase catalyzes elastin degradation and absent inhibition is responsible for emphysema.

Alpha$_1$-antitrypsin irreversibly inactivates neutrophil elastase, but increased neutrophil elastase activity in α_1-antitrypsin-deficient individuals results in matrix destruction. In smokers, significantly increased numbers of neutrophils and amounts of neutrophil elastase within the lung increase the imbalance between proteases and antiproteases. Oxidants in cigarette smoke further decrease α_1-antitrypsin inactivation of neutrophil elastase.

It is postulated that infections trigger an immune response and increased α_1-antitrypsin synthesis in hepatocytes. However, because it cannot be secreted correctly, the abnormal PI Z protein is retained as inclusions within the endoplasmic reticulum of liver cells, leading to inflammation and cirrhosis.

Secretion of PI S protein is similarly impaired and is degraded within the hepatocyte. PI SS homozygotes are not more likely to develop COPD, but PI SZ or PI S with a null allele are associated with an increased risk.

Diagnosis

If serum levels of α_1-antitrypsin are below 11 μmol/L, PCR can be used to determine whether the PI Z allele is present. If it is not, genomic analysis can detect other mutant alleles.

Counselling issues

Alpha$_1$-antitrypsin deficiency has been shown to have adverse psychological effects. Many patients retire early or move to less physically demanding jobs. Exogenous α_1-antitrypsin is available for patients with severe disease.

Related conditions

Patients with mutations in the 3′ flanking sequence of the *PI* gene also have an increased risk of COPD, although they have normal *PI* genes and normal levels of α_1-antitrypsin. It has been postulated that the mutation causes reduced synthesis of α_1-antitrypsin in response to interleukin 6 (IL-6) during inflammation, blocking the normal physiological defense against proteolysis during inflammation in the lung.

References

Anonymous. Alpha$_1$-antitrypsin deficiency: memorandum from a WHO meeting. Bull World Health Organ 1997;75:397–415.

Mahadeva R. Lomas DA. Genetics and respiratory disease. 2. Alpha$_1$-antitrypsin deficiency, cirrhosis and emphysema. Thorax 1998;53:501–5.

Stoller JK. Clinical features and natural history of severe α_1-antitrypsin deficiency. Chest 1997;111:123S–128S.

Chronic Obstructive Pulmonary Disease

(also known as: COPD)

MIM 130700

Clinical features COPD can be divided into 2 diseases: chronic bronchitis and emphysema. Patients with chronic bronchitis have a productive cough, with greater mucus production in the morning, which becomes worse during acute exacerbations. Emphysema is an anatomical description of distal airway enlargement with alveolar destruction and resultant loss of elastic recoil. Wheezing is prominent due to partially reversible airway obstruction and distal airway inflammation. Dyspnea on exertion, hypercapnia, clubbing, and pulmonary hypertension may develop over time. Hemoptysis can occur, but may also reflect underlying lung carcinoma. Physical examination reveals pursed lip expiration, wheezing, prolonged expiration, flattened diaphragms, hyperinflation, and increased chest diameter. Chest X-ray shows a long, narrow heart, flattened diaphragms, areas of hyperlucency, and bullae. Pulmonary function testing demonstrates decreased FEV1 and D_LCO with increased TLC, FRC, and RV (residual volume).

Age of onset Adulthood

Epidemiology About 14 million Americans have COPD. Men are more often affected than women. Mortality is highest in whites and inversely related to socioeconomic status.

Inheritance Deficiencies of α_1-antitrypsin and α_1-antichymotrypsin can cause COPD, but most cases are thought to reflect polygenic and environmental influences.

Genes Data regarding genes involved in the pathogenesis of COPD are inconsistent. Table 2 lists some genes shown to be associated. It should be noted that study results for most genes listed are conflicting, which may reflect the different influences of a gene in different populations.

Gene	Locus	Variants	Disease risk	Functional significance
Glutathione S-transferase M1 (GSTM1)	1p13.3	Homozygous deletion of entire gene	Greater odds of emphysema	Patients with COPD have increased production of reactive oxygen species, levels of which can be regulated by glutathione S-transferases. Deficiency of GSTM1 could lead to increased oxidative damage
Microsomal epoxide hydrolase (mEPHX)	1q42.1	His^{113}/His^{139}	Greater odds of COPD and emphysema	mEPHX detoxifies harmful epoxides found in tobacco smoke. This haplotype results in low enzymatic activity
Cytochrome P450IA1	15q22–q24	$I^{462}V$	Greater odds of centriacinar emphysema	P450 cytochromes detoxify polyaromatic hydrocarbons found in tobacco smoke, but can create toxic products. This polymorphism increases activity of the cytochrome
TNF-α	6p21.3	-308G/A	Greater odds of chronic bronchitis	This polymorphism in the promoter region increases expression of TNF-α, which enhances lung inflammation
Blood group A	9q34		Greater odds of COPD and more rapid decline of lung function	Most individuals secrete blood group antigens into the respiratory tract. It is postulated that the antigens affect microbial defense, although evidence is not conclusive
Vitamin D binding protein (VDBP)	4q12	Gc2, Gc1F	Lower odds of COPD	VDBP may be converted into a macrophage-activating factor (MAF). The Gc2 allele side chain could alter its conversion to an MAF, reducing macrophage-mediated inflammation

Table 2. Partial list of genes that have been associated with disease risk or severity.

Diagnosis

Chronic bronchitis is defined as a chronic, productive cough for at least 3 months per year over 2 consecutive years. Although emphysema is an anatomic diagnosis, it is usually made clinically on the basis of smoking history, presence of wheezing and dyspnea, prolonged expiration, hyperinflation, and spirometry.

Counselling Issues

Smoking is the most significant risk factor for COPD. Patients are at an increased risk of lung carcinoma even after controlling for smoking history.

References

Barnes PJ. Genetics and pulmonary medicine. 9. Molecular genetics of chronic obstructive pulmonary disease. Thorax 1999;54:245–52.

Sandford AJ, Pare PD. Genetic risk factors for chronic obstructive pulmonary disease. Clin Chest Med 2000;21:633–43.

Congenital Alveolar Proteinosis

(also known as: Pulmonary alveolar proteinosis)

MIM 265120

Clinical features Infants can develop persistent pulmonary hypertension, bronchopulmonary dysplasia, and death from respiratory failure. Severe respiratory distress may require mechanical ventilation and extracorporeal membrane oxygenation.

Age of onset Infancy, often within hours of birth.

Epidemiology Rare

Inheritance Autosomal recessive

Chromosomal location *PSP-B*; 2p12–p11.2
CSF2RB; 22q12.2–q13.1

Genes Mutations have been mapped to two genes. *PSP-B*, encoding the pulmonary surfactant protein B on chromosome 2, spans eleven exons over 9.5 kb. The gene product is a hydrophobic protein that transports phospholipids to the air-surface interface, reducing surface tension in alveoli. The *CSF2RB* gene on chromosome 22 encodes the 897-amino acid β chain shared by the granulocyte-macrophage colony-stimulating factor (GM-CSF), interleukin (IL)-3, and IL-5 receptors. The common β chain dimerizes with a specific α chain to create unique receptors with high affinity for GM-CSF, IL-3, or IL-5.

Mutational spectrum The most common *PSP-B* gene defect is a frameshift mutation (121ins2). A proline to threonine change at codon 602 (P602T) is the only identified mutation in the GM-CSF/IL-3/IL-5 receptor common β chain.

Effect of mutation

Absence of transport of phospholipids to the air-surface layer in alveoli has been observed in surfactant protein (SP)-B deficiency, but it is unclear how this contributes to the characteristic histology. A defect in the common β chain might interfere with normal clearance of surfactant proteins by alveolar macrophages.

Diagnosis

Diagnosis is made based upon the presence of eosinophilic, diastase-resistant, periodic acid-Schiff staining granular material with foamy alveolar macrophages and desquamated epithelial cells in alveoli on open-lung biopsy. SP-B in bronchiolar lavage fluid can be assayed using enzyme-linked immunosorbent assay (ELISA), but this test is often not diagnostic.

Counselling issues

There is no effective treatment. Death often occurs early in infancy, but patients with milder disease can live into their teens. Usually, a diagnosis is not made until a second child is afflicted and a biopsy is performed. It is thought that there are additional genes that can cause CAP. Disease may present in adulthood in a form that is idiopathic or associated with viral infection, hematologic malignancy, or lymphoma.

References

Nogee LM, de Mello DE, Dehner LP, et al. Deficiency of pulmonary surfactant protein B in congenital alveolar proteinosis. N Engl J Med 1993;328:406–10.

Nogee LM, Garnier G, Dietz HC, et al. A mutation in the surfactant protein B gene responsible for fatal neonatal respiratory disease in multiple kindreds. J Clin Invest 1994;93:1860–3.

Dirksen U, Nishinakamura R, Groneck P, et al. Human pulmonary alveolar proteinosis associated with a defect in GM-CSF/IL-3/IL-5 receptor common beta chain expression. J Clin Invest 1997;100:2211–2217.

Cutis Laxa

(also known as: Generalized elastolysis)

MIM	219100
Clinical features	Shortness of breath, cough, obstructive pattern on pulmonary function tests, and bullae and hyperinflation on chest X-ray are characteristic of pulmonary emphysema. Clinical features include generalized skin laxity, joint hypermobility, prominent veins, hiatal and other hernias, pre- or post-natal growth restriction, motor development delay, large ears, hooked nose, Wormian bones in the lambdoid sutures, multiple gastrointestinal diverticula, and obstructive uropathy.
Age of onset	Birth, but pulmonary symptoms appear only in the fourth to sixth decades.
Epidemiology	Rare
Inheritance	Autosomal recessive
Chromosomal location	5q23.3–q31.2
Genes	Lysyl oxidase, a 417-amino acid, 32-kD protein encoded by the *LOX* gene, is transcribed as a proproenzyme, but, after N-glycosylation and signal sequence cleavage, it is secreted into the extracellular matrix as a proenzyme which is converted by a metalloproteinase to form the functioning enzyme. Lysyl oxidase, with copper as a cofactor, catalyzes the oxidation of peptidyl lysine to a peptidyl aldehyde, which can condense with other aldehydes or neighboring amino acids to create covalent crosslinks required for maturation of collagen and elastin.
Mutational spectrum	No specific mutations have been identified.

Effect of mutation

It is unknown how the mutations cause disease. In one study, steady state levels of mRNA were not different from controls, indicating that cleavage of the proproenzyme or proenzyme might be the problem.

Diagnosis

Diagnosis is supported by low levels of lysyl oxidase activity in skin fibroblasts with normal levels of serum copper and ceruloplasmin, in the presence of characteristic signs and symptoms.

Counselling

Most patients undergo multiple gastrointestinal or gynecologic surgeries for the management of hernias and rectal or uterine prolapse, and many have plastic surgery to remove excess loose skin.

There are other autosomal dominant (MIM 123700) and X-linked (MIM 304150) forms of the disease that usually lack pulmonary manifestations. The former is due to mutations in the elastin gene on chromosome 7, whereas the latter, also known as Menkes' syndrome, is due to a mutation in an ATP-dependent copper transporter.

References

Khakoo A, Thomas R, Trompeter R, et al. Congenital cutis laxa and lysyl oxidase deficiency. Clin Genet 1997;51:109–14.

Smith-Mungo LI, Kagan HM. Lysyl oxidase: properties, regulation and multiple functions in biology. Matrix Biol 1998;16:387–98.

Fabry's disease

(also known as: Angiokeratoma corporis diffusum; Alpha-galactosidase A deficiency; Anderson-Fabry disease; Hereditary dystopic lipidosis)

MIM 301500

Clinical features Pulmonary symptomatology includes cough, dyspnea on exertion, wheezing, pneumothorax, and an obstructive pattern seen on pulmonary function tests. Patients may have multiple angiokeratomas especially on the inner thighs and groin, hypohidrosis and heat intolerance, acroparesthesias, low-grade fever, autonomic dysfunction, thrombotic events, and ocular disorders. Cardiac involvement results in arrhythmias, angina, and left ventricular hypertrophy. Progression to renal failure and stroke can occur.

Age of onset Mid-childhood

Epidemiology 1:117 000

Inheritance X-linked recessive

Chromosomal location Xq22

Genes The seven-exon *GLA* gene encodes lysosomal α-galactosidase, a 50-kD protein that exists as a homodimer and cleaves an α-galactosyl bond in globotriaosylceramide.

Mutational spectrum Missense mutations are most common, but nonsense, splice-site, and gene rearrangements are also noted. Mutations are usually unique to each family, but $N^{215}S$, $R^{227}Q$, $R^{227}X$, and $R^{342}Q$ have been found in several different families.

Effect of mutation The mutations result in accumulation of globotriaosylceramide primarily in lysosomes of endothelial and smooth muscle cells.

Leukocytes, fibroblasts, and the renal, cardiac, and nervous systems may also be involved.

Diagnosis

Diagnosis is made by mutation analysis of the gene, biochemical assay of α-galactosidase A in leukocytes or fibroblasts, or histopathologic examination of skin or bone marrow that reveals lipid deposition and capillary dilatation.

Counselling issues

Because it is X-linked, Fabry's disease occurs almost exclusively in males. Unequal lyonization of the X-chromosome, however, can cause mild disease in heterozygous females. Patients often die in the sixth decade of renal disease.

References

Brown LK, Miller A, Bhuptani A, et al. Pulmonary involvement in Fabry's disease. Am J Respir Crit Care Med 1997;155:1004–10.

Desnick RJ, Ioannou YA, Eng CM. α-Galactosidase A deficiency: Fabry's disease. In: Scriver CR, Beaudet AL, Sly WS, Valle D, editors. The Metabolic and Molecular Basis of Inherited Disease. 8th ed. New York: McGraw-Hill; 2001. p. 3733–74.

Lysinuric Protein Intolerance

(also known as: Dibasicaminoaciduria II)

MIM	222700
Clinical features	Pulmonary fibrosis, alveolar hemorrhage, and alveolar proteinosis can occur. Other signs and symptoms include postnatal growth restriction, hepatosplenomegaly, severe osteoporosis, anemia, leukopenia, high serum ferritin levels, hypotonia, and mental retardation in the presence of prolonged hyperammonemia.
Age of onset	Onset is often detected by early childhood.
Epidemiology	Disease is rare, with about 100 known cases in the world.
Inheritance	Autosomal recessive
Chromosomal location	14q11.2
Genes	The defect is in the L-type amino acid transporter I *SLC7A7*, which heterodimerizes with another cell surface protein, 4F2 heavy chain (4F2hc), to allow transit of lysine, arginine, and ornithine across the basolateral membrane of epithelial cells.
Mutational spectrum	The most common mutation is a 10-bp deletion beginning at nucleotide 1181, but others include substitution, premature termination, and frameshifts.
Effect of mutation	Deficiencies of lysine, arginine, and ornithine occur due to decreased intestinal absorption and increased renal tubular excretion. Epithelial cells in the liver are unable to secrete these amino acids from the cytoplasm, resulting in intracellular accumulation. Deficiency of ornithine, which is a substrate for ornithine transcarbamylase in the urea cycle, can precipitate hyperammonemia.

Diagnosis

Demonstration of increased urinary excretion of lysine, arginine, and ornithine assists with diagnosis. Serum lysine concentrations are usually less than 80 μmol/L, arginine less than 40 μmol/L, and ornithine less than 20 μmol/L. Serum ammonia levels are increased after an oral or IV protein load. Sequence analysis of genomic DNA is confirmatory.

Counselling issues

Disease prevalence is higher in Finland. There is also a cohort of patients in Naples, Italy. Other cases are sporadic.

References

Parto K, Svedstrom E, Majurin ML, et al. Pulmonary manifestations in lysinuric protein intolerance. Chest 1993;104:1176–82.

Sperandeo MP, Bassi MT, Riboni M, et al. Structure of the SLC7A7 gene and mutational analysis of patients affected by lysinuric protein intolerance. Am J Hum Genet 2000;66:92–9.

Neonatal Respiratory Distress Syndrome

(also known as: Respiratory distress syndrome (RDS); Hyaline membrane disease)

MIM 267450

Clinical features Symptoms include tachypnea, grunting, intercostal retractions, nasal flaring, cyanosis, and apnea. Chest examination can reveal tubular breath sounds with deep inspiratory crackles, most often in the lower lobes. Infants can develop mixed respiratory/metabolic acidosis, oliguria, and ileus.

Age of onset Birth

Epidemiology Incidence is higher in premature infants, but the disease can be present in full-term infants.

Inheritance Autosomal dominant?

Chromosomal location 10q22.2–23.1

Genes Genes for the surfactant proteins A1 (SP-A1) and A2 (SP-A2), located in the same region of chromosome 10, each contain four coding exons and possibly share the same regulatory elements. SP-A1 and SP-A2 are variably altered to create several protein products. Both proteins participate in local host defense and inflammatory responses and counteract dysfunction caused by surfactant inhibitors.

Mutational spectrum Alleles for SP-A1 are designated as 6A(n), whereas SP-A2 alleles are 1A(n). 6A2 homozygosity increases susceptibility to RDS, whereas 6A3 homozygosity is protective. The 6A2/1A0 haplotype may increase susceptibility to RDS.

Effect of mutation 6A2/1A0 haplotypes have lower than normal SP-A1 mRNA levels. It is postulated that this results in deficiency of SP-A1 with disruption of the balance between surfactant and surfactant inhibitors in developing alveoli. The lower effective surfactant concentration means greater alveolar surface tension at the air-fluid interface.

Diagnosis

Diagnosis can be made clinically by the presence of a fine reticular pattern with air-bronchograms on chest X-ray, disturbances of acid-base balance, hypoxemia, and hypercarbia.

Counselling issues

Prematurity greatly increases the chance of neonatal respiratory distress syndrome. There are also many other unknown factors that can affect the incidence of the disease.

References

Ramet M, Haataja R, Marttila R, et al. Association between the surfactant protein A (SP-A) gene locus and respiratory-distress syndrome in the Finnish population. Am J Hum Genet 2000;66:1569–79.

Flores J, Kala P. Surfactant proteins: Molecular genetics and neonatal pulmonary diseases. Annu Rev Physiol 1998;60:365–84.

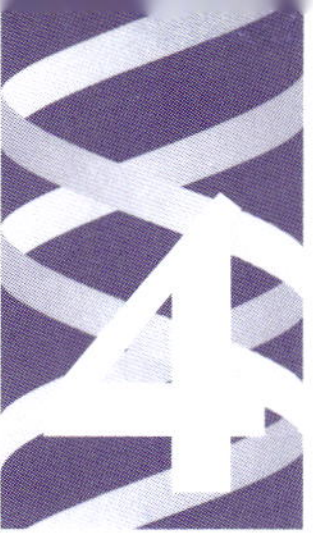

4. Infiltrative lung disorders

Farber's lipogranulomatosis 62

Gaucher's disease 65

Globoid cell leukodystrophy 69

Niemann-Pick disease types A and B 71

Niemann-Pick disease type C 74

Farber's Lipogranulomatosis

(also known as: Farber's disease; Ceramidase deficiency)

MIM 228000

Clinical features

Seven types of Farber's lipogranulomatosis have been categorized, but only types 1 and 4 have lung involvement.

Type 1, Classic

Pulmonary infiltrates and obstructive respiratory insufficiency develop due to granuloma formation and swelling of the larynx and epiglottis. Patients have arthritis of the elbow, knee, wrist, ankle, metacarpophalangeal (MCP), proximal interphalangeal (PIP), or distal interphalangeal (DIP) joints with subcutaneous nodules over affected joints and pressure areas. Patients may also develop hypotonia and muscle atrophy, hepatomegaly, and various abnormalities in the central nervous system.

Type 4, Neonatal Visceral

This type has been reported very rarely and includes extreme histiocytic infiltration of the lungs, causing respiratory insufficiency, and other organs, including the liver, spleen, and thymus. Individuals with Type 4 differ from Type 1 in that they do not develop arthritis, subcutaneous nodules, or laryngeal involvement.

Age of onset Manifestations appear within weeks to months of birth.

Epidemiology Fewer than 50 cases have been reported.

Inheritance Autosomal recessive

Chromosomal location 8p22–p21.3

Genes

Acid ceramidase, a 395-amino acid, 44-kD lysosomal protein, functions in sphingolipid metabolism by degrading ceramide into a fatty acid and a long-chain base, usually sphingosine. Alkaline and neutral ceramidases are unaffected in this disease.

Mutational spectrum

Three missense mutations ($M^{72}V$, $I^{92}V$, and $T^{222}K$) have been identified, all in one patient with Type 1.

Effect of mutation

A deficiency of acid ceramidase leads to accumulation of ceramide in tissues, which causes granulomata and histiocytic infiltration, although the mechanism is not fully understood. Ceramide functions as part of the barrier in normal skin, and although there is ceramide metabolism in the bone marrow and reticuloendothelial cells, these tissues are not affected. It has been postulated that alkaline or neutral ceramidases may be more active at these sites and compensate for the absence of acid ceramidase. It is thought that ceramide accumulation might also affect apoptosis, cell differentiation, and signaling by tumor necrosis factor (TNF)-α, interleukin (IL)-1, and other growth factors, since ceramide functions in all these pathways.

Diagnosis

The classic triad of subcutaneous nodules, arthritis, and laryngeal abnormalities is virtually diagnostic. Low ceramidase activity can be demonstrated *in vitro* in cultured fibroblasts, amniocytes, or leukocytes. Diagnosis can also be established by the presence of granulomata and macrophages with the typical lipid cytoplasmic pattern in a subcutaneous nodule biopsy. Ceramide levels can be measured in various body tissues and fluids.

Counselling issues

There is no effective therapy and patients usually die by age 1–2 years. Prenatal diagnosis can be made using amniocytes or chorionic villus sampling.

References

Koch J. Molecular cloning and characterization of a full-length complementary DNA encoding human acid ceramidase. Identification of the first molecular lesion causing Farber disease. J Biol Chem 1996;271:33110–5.

Moser HW. Acid ceramidase deficiency: Farber lipogranulomatosis. In: Scriver CR, Beaudet AL, Sly WS, Valle D, editors. The Metabolic and Molecular Basis of Inherited Disease. 8th ed. New York: McGraw-Hill; 2001. p. 3573–88.

Gaucher's Disease

(also known as: Glucocerebrosidase deficiency; β-glucosidase deficiency)

Type I

(also known as: GD 1; Gaucher's disease, nonneuronopathic; Gaucher's disease, noncerebral juvenile; Gaucher's disease, adult)

Type II

(also known as: GD 2; Gaucher's disease, acute neuronopathic; Gaucher's disease, infantile cerebral)

Type III

(also known as: GD 3; Gaucher's disease, subacute neuronopathic; Gaucher's disease, cerebral juvenile and adult; Gaucher's Norrbottnian disease)

MIM

230800 Type I
230900 Type II
231000 Type III

Clinical features

Type I

Pulmonary involvement, including interstitial or alveolar infiltration by Gaucher cells, is rare, but is associated with more severe disease. Patients can develop pulmonary hypertension, intrapulmonary right-to-left shunts, or fatal respiratory infections. Gaucher cells, the pathognomonic histologic sign of the disease, are lipid-laden macrophages that collect in the liver, spleen, bone marrow, and bone, causing thrombocytopenia, anemia, hepatosplenomegaly, the classic "Erlenmeyer flask deformity" of the distal femur on X-ray, and painful bone crises. Hematologic malignancies are more common in these patients.

Type II

Unlike Type I, Type II exhibits neurologic manifestations as an important component. Bulbar motor impairment results in dysphagia, aspiration, and fatal pneumonia. Extensive Gaucher cell infiltration of alveoli and alveolar capillaries is often present. The first signs may be ophthalmologic and include bilateral strabismus or oculomotor apraxia. Seizures, spastic limbs, and hypertonic neck musculature are also seen. Hepatosplenomegaly, lymphadenopathy, and other visceral organ involvement are more pronounced than in Type I.

Type III

This is similar to Type II, except that it progresses slowly and is less severe. Dyspnea on exertion and tachypnea due to hepatosplenomegaly are common. Reticular nodular patterns are occasionally seen on chest X-ray. Neurologic manifestations, especially ocular gaze palsies, usually manifest later.

Age of onset

The onset of Type I is in the third to fifth decade, although some subjects may never come to medical attention. Type II is diagnosed in infancy, whereas Type III manifests later in infancy or childhood.

Epidemiology

The incidence is 1:800–4000 in Ashkenazi Jews, and 1:50 000–75 000 in other populations.

Inheritance

Autosomal recessive

Chromosomal location

1q21

Genes

Glucocerebrosidase, an enzyme in the degradation pathway of most glycosphingolipids, catalyzes the conversion of glucosylceramide to ceramide and glucose. The gene spans 7 kb with 11 exons. A 5-kb pseudogene located 16 kb downstream is highly homologous to the functional gene.

Mutational spectrum

Three common mutations comprise up to 95% of the disease-causing alleles in Ashkenazi Jews. These are an asparagine to serine mutation at amino acid 370 ($N^{370}S$), a guanine insertion at nucleotide 84 causing a premature stop codon, and proline replacement of leucine at codon 444 ($L^{444}P$). A common haplotype due to three single base pair mutations, $L^{444}P/A^{456}P/V^{460}V$, known as the recombinant allele, is identical to a region in exon 10 of the pseudogene. More than 50 mutations have been described.

Effect of mutation

All known mutations result in proteins with lower activity or greater instability of glucocerebrosidase, leading to an increase in glucosylceramide. Several genotype/phenotype correlations have been made. The $N^{370}S$/other mutation haplotypes are a cause of Type I, the combination of $L^{444}P$ and the recombinant allele have been implicated in Type II, and $L^{444}P$ homozygotes develop Type III. Certain mutations (e.g. recombinant allele homozygosity) result in fetal or neonatal death.

Diagnosis

Diagnosis is traditionally made by the presence of Gaucher cells on light microscopy. Enzymatic activity of leukocytes or cultured skin fibroblasts can be used to assess glucocerebrosidase activity. Diagnosis is now made by DNA identification of mutations. Initial screens can be made of the alleles common in Jewish or non-Jewish patients.

Counselling issues

Life expectancy differs based on disease type. Type I patients have lived more than 80 years, whereas Type II patients rarely live past 2 years of age, and Type III patients survive into their 30's. Recombinant glucocerebrosidase is commercially available for replacement therapy. Because of susceptibility to fractures and slow healing, some physicians recommend only non-contact sports or activities. Carrier status can be assessed with screening for the most common mutations, and prenatal diagnosis can be made by amniocentesis.

Related conditions

Two patients with Gaucher's disease and normal glucocerebrosidase activity were found to have a mutation in saposin C (MIM 176801), a cohydrolase needed for proper functioning of glucocerebrosidase.

References

Beutler E, Grabowski GA. Gaucher disease. In: Scriver CR, Beaudet AL, Sly WS, Valle D, editors. The Metabolic and Molecular Basis of Inherited Disease. 8th ed. New York: McGraw-Hill; 2001. p. 3635–68.

Santamaria F, Parenti G, Guidi G, et al. Pulmonary manifestations of

Gaucher disease: an increased risk for L444P homozygotes? Am J Respir Crit Care Med 1998;157:985–89.

Kerem E, Elstein D, Abrahamov A, et al. Pulmonary function abnormalities in type I Gaucher disease. Eur Respir J 1996; 9:340–5.

Globoid Cell Leukodystrophy

(also known as: Krabbe's disease; Galactocerebrosidase deficiency; GLD)

MIM 245200

Clinical features The globoid cell, a derivative of the monocyte-macrophage lineage that is typically found near blood vessels within the central nervous system, is pathognomonic for this disease. Patients can also develop infiltration of alveoli and alveolar ducts with large macrophage-like cells containing intensely eosinophilic cytoplasmic inclusions or multinucleated giant cells. Neurologic abnormalities are marked, with hyperirritability, hypersensitivity to external stimuli, seizures, intellectual and developmental regression, hypertonia, hyperactive reflexes or areflexia, optic atrophy leading to blindness, and eventual progression to a decerebrate condition.

Age of onset Onset is within 1 year of birth.

Epidemiology 1:200 000

Inheritance Autosomal recessive

Chromosomal location 14q31

Genes The gene responsible for globoid cell leukodystrophy, *GALC*, encompassing 56 kb with 17 exons, encodes galactocerebrosidase, a 669-amino acid protein that is cleaved into 50–52-kD and 30-kD subunits, both of which are necessary for activity. Galactocerebrosidase is a lysosomal enzyme that degrades galactosylceramide, a glycolipid concentrated in myelin and oligodendrocytes, into galactose and ceramide. Galactocerebrosidase also functions in the degradation of psychosine, monogalactosyldiglyceride, and lactosylceramide.

Mutational spectrum

Whereas most mutations are missense, the mutation 502T/del is responsible for about 50% of all cases in individuals from northern Europe, the United States, and Mexico. It is a 30-kb deletion that begins in intron 10 and leads to absence of the entire 30-kD subunit and part of the 50–52-kD subunit.

Effect of mutation

The mutation causes absence of degradation of galactosylceramide in the white matter of the central nervous system, prompting infiltration by globoid cells. As more galactosylceramide accumulates, oligodendrocytes undergo apoptosis and the process of myelination is disrupted. In addition, the level of psychosine, which is known to be toxic to oligodendrocytes, increases up to 100-fold. The absence of oligodendrocytes and myelin results in neurologic abnormalities. The origin of the cells that infiltrate the respiratory system is unclear.

Diagnosis

The usual method of diagnosis is to assay galactocerebrosidase activity in leukocytes or cultured fibroblasts. Analysis of the genomic DNA sequence can be used for confirmation.

Counselling issues

Death by 3 years of age is usual. Chorionic villus biopsy can be used for prenatal diagnosis of at-risk pregnancies.

Related conditions

There is a late-onset form of the disease, in which most patients develop symptoms by age 10. It is associated with an initial rapid progression of disease, followed by prolonged, slower deterioration.

References

Wenger DA, Rafi MA, Luzi P, et al. Krabbe disease: genetic aspects and progress toward therapy. Mol Genet Metab 2000;70:1–9.

Wenger DA, Suzuki K, Suzuki Y, Suzuki K. Galactosylceramide lipidosis: globoid cell leukodystrophy (Krabbe disease). In: Scriver CR, Beaudet AL, Sly WS, Valle D, editors. The Metabolic and Molecular Basis of Inherited Disease. 8th ed. New York: McGraw-Hill; 2001. p. 3669–94.

Niemann-Pick Disease Types A and B

(also known as: Sphingomyelin lipidosis; Sphingomyelinase deficiency)

MIM

257200

Clinical features

Type A

Feeding difficulties and failure to thrive may be the initial presentation. Infants develop repeated episodes of bronchitis or aspiration pneumonias. Chest X-ray shows a diffuse reticular or fine nodular pattern due to lipid-containing foamy cells infiltrating pulmonary alveoli and septa. Hepatosplenomegaly and a protuberant abdomen are prominent features. Muscle hypotonia and psychomotor retardation progress to spasticity and limited interaction with the environment. The classic sign is a cherry-red spot on the macula.

Type B

Patients have a diffuse reticular pattern on chest X-ray, similar to Type A, but suffer from more severe pulmonary infections. Patients approaching their second decade have increasing dyspnea and hypoxia. Splenomegaly becomes relatively less prominent with age as height increases, but splenectomy may be required if pancytopenia develops. Other complications include cirrhosis, portal hypertension, and ascites. Unlike Type A, Type B does not involve neurological or intellectual impairment.

Age of onset

Onset of Type A is within a few months of birth, whereas Type B onset is in infancy or childhood.

Epidemiology

The gene frequency in Ashkenazi Jews is 1:200 for Type A and 1:400 for Type B. The prevalence is 1:250 000 in other populations.

Inheritance

Autosomal recessive

Chromosomal location 11p15.4–p15.1

Genes

The *SMPD1* gene contains six exons ranging in size from 77 to 773 kb, with exon 2 encoding 44% of the total protein. It encodes the 70-kD acid sphingomyelinase, which is localized to the lysosomal membrane in liver, brain, placenta, and kidney and is responsible for cleaving sphingomyelin into ceramide and phosphocholine. Sphingomyelin, a phospholipid component of the cell membrane, endoplasmic reticulum, mitochondria, and other subcellular organelles, is especially abundant in myelin cells.

Mutational spectrum

Twelve mutations have been identified. The three most common are the point mutations $R^{496}L$ and $L^{302}P$, and a single base deletion leading to a premature stop codon at codon 330.

Effect of mutation

Type A

These mutations yield an enzyme with almost no catalytic activity, causing abnormal cell membrane turnover and accumulation of sphingomyelin. Cholesterol and bis(monoacylglycero)phosphate also accumulate, presumably due to lipid-lipid interactions in cell membranes and the increased number of lysosomes, respectively. Reticuloendothelial cells, mostly in the spleen and lymph nodes but also in the lung, kidney, liver, and brain, phagocytose the excess sphingomyelin and cholesterol.

Type B

Patients with Type B have one allele encoding an enzyme with no catalytic activity and another yielding a protein with minimal activity, resulting in a total activity 2–10% of normal, which is sufficient to prevent neurologic manifestations.

Diagnosis

Acid sphingomyelinase activity can be measured in cultured fibroblasts, leukocytes, or lymphoblasts. Sphingomyelin levels can also be assayed and are usually increased 2–50-fold. The three most common mutations can be identified by a PCR-based analysis of DNA.

Counselling issues

Prenatal diagnosis can be established by measuring acid sphingomyelinase activity of amniocytes. Type A patients die in early childhood, whereas Type B patients can survive into early adulthood.

Related conditions

Foamy cells are also found in patients with GM1 gangliosidosis (MIM 230500), Wolman disease (MIM 278000), and lipoprotein lipase deficiency (MIM 238600).

References

Schuchman EH, Desnick RJ. Niemann-Pick Disease Types A and B: Acid sphingomyelinase deficiencies. In: Scriver CR, Beaudet AL, Sly WS, Valle D, editors. The Metabolic and Molecular Basis of Inherited Disease. 8th ed. New York: McGraw-Hill; 2001. p. 3611–33.

Niemann-Pick Disease Type C

(also known as: Niemann-Pick disease, subacute juvenile form; Niemann-Pick disease, chronic neuronopathic form)

MIM 257220

Clinical features Type C has a heterogenous presentation. Patients have histiocytic infiltration in various organs, including the lungs. Self-limiting neonatal jaundice is present in half of the cases, but hepatosplenomegaly is not as severe as in other forms of Niemann-Pick disease. Vertical supranuclear ophthalmoplegia is manifest in almost all patients. Ataxia, dysphasia, drooling, and dysarthria eventually progress to severe dystonia, cataplexy, and seizures, leaving the patient wheelchair-bound. Severe dysphagia usually leads to death by aspiration. A late-onset phenotype is characterized by more prominent psychiatric disease and intellectual impairment.

Age of onset Onset is usually in childhood, but occurs rarely in adulthood.

Epidemiology 1:200 000

Inheritance Autosomal recessive

Chromosomal location 18q11–q12

Genes *NPC1*, a 47-kb gene with 25 exons, encodes a 1278-amino acid, 142-kD protein. The NPC1 protein is one of a class of membrane-bound proteins with sterol-sensing properties, postulated to be involved in the regulation of intracellular cholesterol through lipid trafficking within the endosomal system.

Mutational spectrum Of ten mutations identified, most are single amino acid substitutions. A more severe form of the disease was noted in patients with a 227-bp deletion in exon 9.

Effect of mutation

The mutations, by a mechanism that remains to be fully elucidated, cause excessive accumulation of LDL-derived cholesterol of lysosomes, especially in presynaptic glial cells in the CNS. The adult-onset form may be due to a combination of the $V^{889}M$ mutation in one allele with the splice site deletion 3043-2delA, resulting in the absence of 18 amino acids downstream.

Diagnosis

Diagnosis is based on the demonstration of diminished cholesterol esterification and perinuclear cholesterol accumulation in filipin-stained cultured fibroblasts.

Counselling issues

Patients benefit from speech, occupational, and physical therapy. Most die between the ages of 5 and 15 years, but those with the adult-onset form may live into the fifth decade. Prenatal diagnosis is established by amniocentesis or chorionic villus sampling.

References

Patterson MC, Vanier MT, Suzuki K, et al. Niemann-Pick disease Type C: A lipid trafficking disorder. In: Scriver CR, Beaudet AL, Sly WS, Valle D, editors. The Metabolic and Molecular Basis of Inherited Disease. 8th ed. New York: McGraw-Hill; 2001. p. 3611–33.

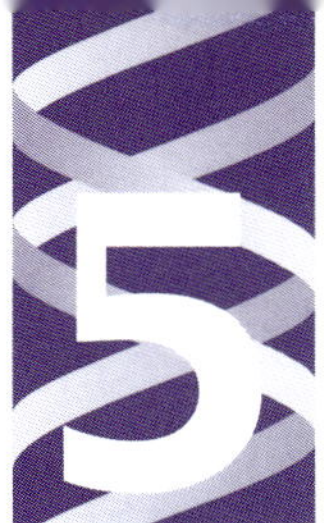

5. Interstitial lung disorders

Ankylosing spondylitis **78**

Dyskeratosis congenita **81**

Familial amyloidosis **83**

Familial interstitial lung disease **85**

Hermansky-Pudlak syndrome **87**

Ankylosing Spondylitis (AS)

(also known as: Marie-Strumpell spondylitis; Bechterew's syndrome)

MIM 106300

Clinical features Pulmonary abnormalities, best seen on CT scan, include pulmonary fibrosis and other nonspecific interstitial changes most often in the upper lobes, bronchiectasis, tracheobronchomegaly, mycetoma formation, aspergillomas, pleural effusions, and pneumothoraces. Cricoarytenoid arthritis, causing upper airway obstruction, has also been reported. Pulmonary function tests usually show a restrictive defect due to costovertebral ankylosis. Characteristic manifestations include sacroiliitis causing low back pain not relieved by rest, limitation of lumbar spine movement, enthesopathy, peripheral arthritis, uveitis, heart conduction defects, and aortitis.

Age of onset Early adulthood

Epidemiology The estimated prevalence is 2–20:10 000 in whites, but lower in Africans and Asians. Prevalence in males is between two and ten times more than in females.

Inheritance Autosomal dominant with variable penetrance

Chromosomal location 6p21.3

Genes HLA-B27, a 359-amino acid protein, is one of the major histocompatibility complex (MHC) class I molecules that present antigens to the T cell receptor on CD8+ cells. MHC class I molecules are heterodimers composed of a 44-kD heavy chain noncovalently associated with a 12-kD light chain. The extracellular portion has a groove containing six pockets involved in binding peptide antigens.

Mutational spectrum

Ten of the 12 different subtypes of HLA-B27 are associated with disease. Prevalence of subtypes varies with ethnicity and geographic locale.

Effect of mutation

Several hypotheses have been proposed to explain the role of HLA-B27 in disease, but the "arthritogenic peptide theory" is currently favored. According to this theory, HLA-B27 preferentially binds host joint-specific peptides due to the 3-dimensional nature of the HLA-B27 binding cleft. Normally, very few circulating T cells recognize this epitope so autoinflammation is not induced. Some bacterial antigens, such as those from *Yersinia*, *Salmonella*, *Shigella*, *Campylobacter*, or *Chlamydia trachomatis*, have peptide motifs similar to joint-specific antigens. Therefore, an infection can increase the number of autoreactive T cells that induce joint inflammation. An alternative theory, "molecular mimicry", states that HLA-B27 is the self-antigen that cross-reacts with the bacterial peptides, inducing autoinflammation.

Diagnosis

The modified New York Criteria for definite diagnosis of AS require either unilateral grade 3 or 4 or bilateral grade 2–4 sacroiliitis, and any of the following clinical criteria:

- lower back pain of at least 3 months duration improved by exercise and not relieved by rest
- limitation of lumbar spine motion in sagittal and frontal planes
- chest expansion below normal for age and sex

Counselling issues

There is a 20% risk of a relative who is also HLA-B27 positive developing AS, but no increased risk if the relative is HLA-B27 negative. Postural training helps improve mobility and range of motion in the back. Exercise, especially swimming, helps relieve pain.

About 90% of patients have HLA-B27, an allele found in 5–15% of the white population. However, 95% of those with HLA-B27 do not have disease.

References

Allen RL, Bowness P, McMichael AJ. The role of HLA-B27 in spondyloarthritis. Immunogenetics 1999;50:220–7.

Fenlon HM, Casserly I, Sant SM, et al. Plain radiographs and thoracic high-resolution CT in patients with ankylosing spondylitis. Am J Roentgenol 1997;168:1067–72.

Dyskeratosis Congenita

(also known as: Zinsser-Cole-Engman syndrome; DC; DKC)

MIM	305000
Clinical features	The combination of pulmonary fibrosis with low diffusion capacity of carbon monoxide (D_LCO) and a telangiectatic pulmonary vasculature can lead to hypoxemia and acrocyanosis. *Pneumocystis carinii* pneumonia can develop secondary to generalized immunodeficiency. Some patients develop pulmonary fibrosis and thickened pleura following bone marrow transplantation. Abnormal skin pigmentation, nail dystrophy, and mucosal leukoplakia are the classic triad, but pancytopenia, developmental delay, short stature, and hematologic and solid tissue malignancies may also be present.
Age of onset	Childhood
Epidemiology	Rare
Inheritance	X-linked recessive
Chromosomal location	Xq28
Genes	The *DKC1* gene, encoding dyskerin, contains 15 exons extending over 15 kb. The 57-kD protein contains 514 amino acids and is highly conserved in eukaryotes. It is a nucleolar protein involved in centromere functioning, nucleocytoplasmic trafficking, stability of H/ACA small nucleolar ribonucleoproteins, ribosomal ribonucleic acid (rRNA) transcription, ribosome biosynthesis, and RNA pseudouridylation.
Mutational spectrum	Most mutations are missense. By far the most common is replacement of arginine by valine at codon 353 ($R^{353}V$). A splice-site mutation, a 3 base-pair deletion, and a 2 base-pair deletion have also been identified. Approximately half of all mutations occur in exons 3 or 4.

Effect of mutation

Cells most affected are those with the highest turnover rate, including hematopoietic, skin, and mucosal cells. This is possibly due to altered ribonucleoprotein assembly on the H/ACA domain of telomerase RNA, but the mechanism has not yet been elucidated.

Diagnosis

Diagnosis is confirmed by SSCP followed by DNA sequence analysis.

Counselling issues

Patients usually die from bone marrow failure, pulmonary complications, or malignancy. Some patients live into adulthood but by age 30 years over 90% of patients have bone marrow failure requiring bone marrow transplant.

Related conditions

The Hoyeraal-Hreidarsson syndrome (MIM 300240) is a severe variant of DC that shows the wide spectrum of clinical manifestations created by mutations in *DKC1*. There are also autosomal recessive (MIM 224230) and autosomal dominant (MIM 127550) forms that occur less frequently.

References

Dokal I. Dyskeratosis congenita in all its forms. Br J Haematol 2000;110:768–79.

Knight SW, Heiss NS, Vulliamy TJ, et al. X-linked dyskeratosis congenita is predominantly caused by missense mutations in the DKC1 gene. Am J Hum Genet 1999;65:50–8.

Mitchell JR, Wood E, Collins K. A telomerase component is defective in the human disease dyskeratosis congenita. Nature 1999;402:551–5.

Paul SR, Perez-Atayde A, Williams DA. Interstitial pulmonary disease associated with dyskeratosis congenita. Am J Pediatr Hematol Oncol 1992;14:89–92.

Familial Amyloidosis

(also known as: Familial amyloidotic polyneuropathy; Amyloidosis type I)

MIM 176300

Clinical features Deposition of amyloid in alveolar septa and the pulmonary vasculature appears as a reticulonodular pattern on chest radiography. Patients may report dyspnea, although this is often a result of congestive heart failure secondary to amyloid deposition in the myocardium. Signs and symptoms are due to amyloid infiltration of various tissues, leading to autonomic and peripheral sensorimotor neuropathy, renal failure, cardiac conduction defects, and vitreous humor clouding.

Age of onset Onset occurs in the fourth to eighth decades.

Epidemiology Rare

Inheritance Autosomal dominant

Chromosomal location 18q11.2–q12.1

Genes The *TTR* gene, which encodes transthyretin, contains four exons spanning 7.6 kb. Transthyretin is a 127-amino acid protein which forms a 55-kD tetramer that transports thyroxine and retinol-binding protein in the serum. Each monomer contains eight β-pleated sheets that are characteristic of amyloid fibrils.

Mutational spectrum All mutations, except for the deletion of codon 122, are missense mutations found in exons 2, 3, or 4. The most common is a methionine replacement for valine at codon 30 ($V^{30}M$) that has been found in several ethnic groups.

Effect of mutation The mechanism is unknown. Originally, it was postulated that amino acid substitutions led to a change in protein conformation, but this has not been proven. Other hypotheses include the formation of an abnormal intermediate tertiary structure that results in amyloid fibrils, or the slower degradation of transthyretin allowing more time for amyloid aggregation.

Diagnosis

Congo red staining shows amyloid fibrils in affected tissues. Transthyretin is then assayed by isoelectric focusing to detect for genetic variants. Direct DNA sequencing identifies specific mutations.

Counselling issues

Manifestations (e.g. cardiac involvement) depend on each specific mutation. About 10% of patients with mutations may never have any symptoms. Patients can live up to 15 years after diagnosis, but survival is shorter the earlier the age of diagnosis. Because transthyretin is produced in the liver, definitive therapy is liver transplantation.

Related conditions

Mutations of other genes are known to cause hereditary amyloidoses. These include apolipoprotein A-I (MIM 107680), gelsolin (MIM 137350), fibrinogen A α polypeptide chain (MIM 134820), lysozyme (MIM 153450), cystatin C (MIM 105150), and amyloid β A4 precursor protein (MIM 104760). In addition, Muckle-Wells syndrome (MIM 191900) and familial visceral amyloidosis (MIM 105200), conditions in which the mutated gene is not known, have amyloidosis as a component.

References

Benson MD. Amyloidosis. In: Scriver CR, Beaudet AL, Sly WS, Valle D, editors. The Metabolic and Molecular Basis of Inherited Disease. 8th ed. New York: McGraw-Hill; 2001. p. 5345–78

Smith RRL, Hutchins GM, Moore GW, et al. Type and distribution of pulmonary parenchymal and vascular amyloid. Correlation with cardiac amyloid. Am J Med 1979;66:96–104.

Familial Interstitial Lung Disease

(also known as: Chronic pneumonitis of infancy)

MIM	178620
Clinical features	Presentation may vary from cough to tachypnea. Severe cases have cyanosis and eventually respiratory distress. Milder cases may receive the diagnosis of gastroesophageal reflux disease, and failure to thrive is often noted. Chest X-ray shows increased interstitial markings, and open lung biopsy demonstrates increased mesenchymal cells in the interstitium, lymphocytic infiltration, and occasional accumulations of alveolar macrophages.
Age of onset	Disease is detected within the first year.
Epidemiology	Rare
Inheritance	Autosomal dominant
Chromosomal location	8p21
Genes	*SFTP2* is a 3.4-kb gene that encodes surfactant protein C, an 18.5-kD protein with a 34-amino acid hydrophobic domain that assists surfactant lipids in reducing surface tension at the air-fluid interface in alveoli.
Mutational spectrum	Only one mutation has been found, a donor splice site mutation of the first base of intron 4 (c.460+1G→A).
Effect of mutation	The splice site mutation causes a 37-amino acid deletion in exon 4. It is postulated that the eliminated region is necessary for proper intracellular trafficking of the precursor protein, which either disrupts the transport of wild-type surfactant protein C or increases the degradation of both wild-type and mutant proteins. Accumulation of the protein or its metabolites may cause cell injury and

inflammation, leading to lung damage. Alternatively, deficiency of surfactant protein C may itself have deleterious effects in the lung.

Diagnosis

Histologic examination of lung tissue is necessary for diagnosis.

Counselling issues

It is likely there are many other genes that cause similar disease. Risk of maternal death during pregnancy may be increased.

Related conditions

Certain alleles of surfactant protein A1 and A2 predispose to neonatal respiratory distress syndrome (MIM 267450). Mutations in surfactant protein B cause pulmonary alveolar proteinosis (MIM 265120).

References

Katzenstein ALA, Gordon LP, Oliphant M, et al. Chronic pneumonitis of infancy. A unique form of interstitial lung disease occurring in early childhood. Am J Surg Pathol 1995;19:439–47.

Nogee LM, Dunbar AE III, Wert SE, et al. A mutation in the surfactant protein C gene associated with familial interstitial lung disease. N Engl J Med 2001;344:573–9.

Hermansky-Pudlak Syndrome

(also known as: Delta storage pool disease; HPS)

MIM

203300

Clinical features

Patients develop bronchiectasis and pulmonary fibrosis, with pulmonary function tests showing decrease in forced expiratory volume in 1 second (FEV_1), forced vital capacity (FVC), total lung capacity (TLC), vital capacity (VC), D_LCO. Oxygen saturation at rest is unaffected. Other findings include oculocutaneous albinism, bleeding diathesis, granulomatous colitis, neutropenia, and accumulation of ceroid lipofuscin in lysosomes.

Age of onset

Birth

Epidemiology

The incidence is 1:1800 in Puerto Ricans, and the disease has also been found in a single family in Valais, Switzerland. Rare sporadic cases have been reported.

Inheritance

Autosomal recessive

Chromosomal location

HPS-1; 10q23.1–q23.3
AP3B1; chr. 5
HPS-3; 3q24

Genes

The *HPS-1* gene, with 20 exons spanning 30.5 kb on chromosome 10, encodes a 700-amino acid, 79.3-kD cytosolic protein hypothesized to be involved in the creation or function of intracellular organelles. Mutations in a second gene on chromosome 5, *AP3B1*, encoding the 1,093-amino acid β-3a subunit of adaptor complex 3, also cause disease. Based on mouse models, involvement of other human genes is postulated, but none have been discovered.

Mutational spectrum

The Puerto Rican mutation is a 16-bp deletion in exon 15 of HPS-1. A frameshift mutation at codon 322 is the most prevalent mutation in Europeans. Different mutations have been seen in Irish, Japanese, Ukrainian, and other populations. Two mutations found in *AP3B1* are a 63-bp deletion (nucleotides 1166–1228) and a substitution of G for T at nucleotide 1739.

Effect of mutation

The effect of the *HPS-1* mutations is unknown. The β-3a subunit of adaptor complex 3 is involved in sorting of proteins to lysosomes, causing defective transport of proteins to melanosomes and dense granules in platelets.

Diagnosis

The presence of oculocutaneous albinism along with absence of dense granules in platelets on electron microscopy is pathognomonic for the disease. PCR-based analysis can confirm the 16-bp deletion of *HPS-1* if there is uncertainty. For patients with other mutations in *HPS-1*, SSCP followed by DNA sequence analysis of the exons can be used to diagnose.

Counselling issues

HPS is especially common in Puerto Ricans. Death usually occurs in the fourth or fifth decade due to impaired pulmonary function.

References

Shotelersuk V, Dell'Angelica EC, Hartnell L, et al. A new variant of Hermansky-Pudlak Syndrome due to mutations in a gene responsible for vesicle formation. Am J Med 2000;108:423–7.

Brantly M, Avila NA, Shotelersuk V, et al. Pulmonary function and high-resolution CT findings in patients with an inherited form of pulmonary fibrosis, Hermansky-Pudlak Syndrome, due to mutations in HPS-1. Chest 2000; 117:129–36.

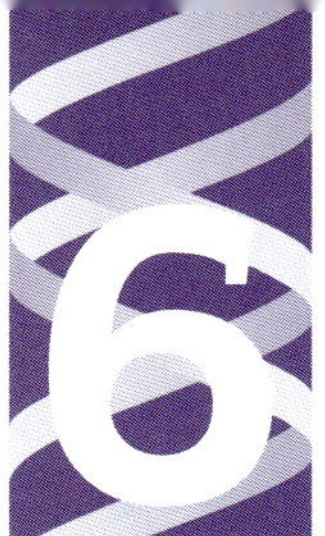

6. Disorders of the vasculature and blood

Hereditary hemorrhagic telangiectasia **90**

Familial primary pulmonary hypertension **92**

Sickle cell disease **94**

Disorders that predispose to pulmonary emboli:

Activated protein C resistance **97**

Antithrombin III deficiency **99**

Dysfibrinogenemia **101**

Hyperhomocysteinemia **103**

Protein C/protein S deficiencies **105**

Prothrombin gene mutation **107**

Hereditary Hemorrhagic Telangiectasia

(also known as: HHT; Osler-Rendu-Weber disease)

MIM	HHT1; 187300 HHT2; 600376
Clinical features	Patients may have extensive pulmonary arteriovenous malformation (AVM) leading to significant right-to-left shunting. Symptoms and signs include dyspnea on exertion, profound hypoxemia, orthodeoxia, hemoptysis, chest pain, cyanosis, bruits, and clubbing. The initial symptom is often epistaxis, occasionally severe enough to require transfusion. Telangiectases may be present in the nasal and oral mucosa, skin, conjunctiva, gastrointestinal tract, and brain. Paradoxical emboli may result in thromboembolic strokes or brain abscesses.
Age of onset	Epistaxis often occurs by age 10 years and cutaneous lesions appear later. Penetrance depends on age and approaches 97% by age 40 years.
Epidemiology	1:10 000–50 000
Inheritance	Autosomal dominant
Chromosomal location	HHT1; 9q34.1 HHT2; 12q11–q14
Genes	*ENG*, also known as *CD105*, is a 14-exon gene on chromosome 9 encoding a protein known as endoglin that is localized to vascular endothelial cells. *ACVRLK1*, on chromosome 12, encodes activin-A receptor type II-like kinase 1 (ALK1), a receptor for the transforming growth factor (TGF)-β superfamily of proteins.
Mutational spectrum	Deletion, nonsense, or missense mutations in *ENG* most often result in truncated proteins or unstable mRNA. For *ACVRLK1*, missense

and deletion mutations result in amino acid substitutions or truncated proteins.

Effect of mutation

It has not been shown how these mutations cause disease. One postulate for both genes is that if one allele is mutated, the normal allele cannot produce enough protein to compensate for the decreased production of the mutant allele, a phenomenon known as haploinsufficiency.

Diagnosis

To establish the diagnosis, patients should have three of the following four clinical characteristics: recurrent spontaneous epistaxis, telangiectases in various locations, visceral organ involvement, and significant family history. Analysis of the two genetic loci should also be completed.

Counselling issues

Mortality from untreated, symptomatic pulmonary AVMs at 15 years after diagnosis is as much as 22%. Pulmonary AVMs are more common in patients with endoglin mutations. Seventy percent of patients who have pulmonary AVMs have HHT. Because of the autosomal dominant inheritance pattern, family members should be screened for disease.

References

Shovlin CL, Letarte M. Hereditary haemorrhagic telangiectasia and pulmonary arteriovenous malformations: issues in clinical management and review of pathogenic mechanisms. Thorax 1999;54:714–29.

Haitjema T, Westermann CJ, Overtoom TT, et al. Hereditary hemorrhagic telangiectasia (Osler-Weber-Rendu disease): new insights in pathogenesis, complications, and treatment. Arch Intern Med 1996;156:714–19.

Familial Primary Pulmonary Hypertension

(also known as: PPH1; PHT; FPPH)

MIM 178600

Clinical features Patients often present with dyspnea on exertion and hypoxemia. Pulmonary function tests are usually normal except for a low diffusion capacity of carbon monoxide (D_LCO). Ventilation/perfusion (V/Q) scan shows normal ventilation but abnormal perfusion, which may reflect thrombo-occlusion. Chest X-ray may show peripheral pulmonary vascular markings, cardiomegaly, and increased prominence of the pulmonary arteries. Elevated pulmonary artery pressure is almost invariably present. Other signs may include elevated jugular venous pressure, right ventricular heave, loud pulmonary component of the second heart sound, pulmonary flow murmur, hepatojugular reflex, hepatic pulsation, and lower extremity edema.

Age of onset Early to middle adulthood

Epidemiology 1–10:1 000 000. Prevalence in females is twice that in males.

Inheritance Autosomal dominant with incomplete penetration

Chromosomal location 2q33

Genes *BMPR2*, the bone morphogenetic protein receptor type 2, is a member of the transforming growth factor receptor superfamily. The gene contains 13 exons, and its 115-kD protein product has 1038 amino acids. The type 2 receptor forms a heterodimer with the type 1 receptor to produce a complex in which the type 2 receptor is necessary for ligand binding while the type 1 receptor is responsible for intracellular signaling.

Mutational spectrum Of the 14 mutations identified, five are missense, five are frameshift, and four are nonsense.

Effect of mutation

Mutations may prevent the protein from associating with or phosphorylating the type 1 receptor. It is hypothesized that, by altering the ability of the type 1 receptor to induce apoptosis in certain cell types, increased cell proliferation results in the development of PPH. Phenotypes are consistent with the models of haploinsufficiency or dominant negative.

All three layers of the arterial wall are affected in PPH. There is increased fibrosis and thickening of the intima, hypertrophy of smooth muscle as well as increased matrix protein and connective tissue in the media, and fibroblast proliferation with resultant additional extracellular matrix deposition in the adventitia. Impaired vasodilatation and enhanced vasoconstriction may occur, perhaps through alterations in the nitric oxide and endothelin 1 pathways.

Diagnosis

Right heart catheterization reveals elevated pulmonary arterial pressures in the absence of a cardiac shunt.

Counselling issues

Median survival is usually 2 years after diagnosis. First-degree relatives should be screened with transthoracic echocardiography when an index case is diagnosed and at any time when symptoms suggestive of pulmonary hypertension develop.

PPH shows "anticipation", meaning that patients in later generations have worse disease. There is also incomplete penetration so that some carriers of the abnormal gene may not be affected.

References

Deng Z, Morse JH, Slager SL, et al. Familial primary pulmonary hypertension (gene PPH1) is caused by mutations in the bone morphogenetic protein receptor-II gene. Am J Hum Genet 2000;67:737–44.

Lane KB, Machado RD, Pauciulo MW, et al. Heterozygous germline mutations in BMPR2, encoding a TGF-beta receptor, cause familial primary pulmonary hypertension. The International PPH Consortium. Nat Genet 2000;26:81–4.

Peacock AJ. Primary pulmonary hypertension. Thorax 1999;54:1107–18.

Sickle Cell Disease

(also known as: Sickle cell anemia)

MIM 603903

Clinical features Patients often develop an acute chest syndrome characterized by pleuritic pain, dyspnea, tachypnea, cough, splinting and atelectasis due to vertebral or rib infarction, hypoxemia, fever, lung crackles on auscultation, and infiltrates on chest X-ray. Pneumonia, frequently due to *Pneumocystis carinii*, viruses, or atypical bacteria, may present in a similar fashion. Some patients develop a chronic lung disease characterized by hypoxemia, a restrictive pattern on pulmonary function tests, and chest X-ray evidence of interstitial fibrosis and cor pulmonale. Hematologic manifestations include sickled erythrocytes, chronic hemolytic anemia, and reticulocytosis. Other abnormalities include diffuse microinfarcts in all organs, functional asplenia, septicemia, stroke, priapism, cholelithiasis, osteomyelitis, ineffective urine concentration, and leg ulcerations.

Age of onset Infancy to childhood

Epidemiology 0.16% of African-Americans

Inheritance Autosomal recessive

Chromosomal location 11p15.5

Genes *HBB*, the hemoglobin β-globin gene, contains 625 bases that encode 147 amino acids. Two α and two β chains combine to form a functional heterotetrameric protein.

Mutational spectrum Most cases are due to the hemoglobin (Hb) S allele, a valine for glutamic acid substitution at position 6 (G^6V). However, when the Hb C allele (G^6K) is heterozygous with Hb S, the phenotype is similar. Disease can occur also when one allele is Hb S and the other is a β-thalassemia mutation. Almost 500 different mutations in the β-globin gene have been identified.

Effect of mutation

Deoxygenated hemoglobin S undergoes a conformational change, resulting in separation of β subunits and allowing the hydrophobic valine in position 6 to bind to a hydrophobic site on a neighboring hemoglobin molecule. When this occurs slowly, aggregation of multiple hemoglobin molecules results in polymers that induce the sickle shape of the erythrocyte. There is also upregulation of adhesion molecules on sickled and unsickled erythrocytes, increased concentration of certain plasma proteins (e.g. von Willebrand factor), decreased concentration of certain coagulation inhibitors, and decreased production of signaling molecules (e.g. nitric oxide). Sickled cells damage the vascular endothelium, contributing to adhesion and trapping of erythrocytes and sickled cells. This cell accumulation, along with a hypercoagulable state, promotes thrombus formation and vascular obstruction.

The acute chest syndrome is thought to be secondary to infarction of the bone marrow, from which fat emboli travel to the pulmonary circulation. Increased concentration of free fatty acids, which promotes platelet aggregation and activation of coagulation factors, may result from the activation of phospholipase A2. In addition, sickled cells and erythrocytes adhere to the pulmonary vascular endothelium. These factors combine to cause pulmonary infarction characteristic of the acute chest syndrome.

Diagnosis

Diagnosis is made by PCR-based identification of the Hb S or Hb C alleles.

Counselling issues

Mortality is highest in the first year of life. Median life expectancy is 42 years for males and 48 for females. In addition to Africans, there are populations in India, Saudi Arabia, and Greece that also have a high frequency of sickle cell disease. Prenatal diagnosis can be made by amniocentesis or chorionic villus sampling.

Hb S heterozygotes who are infected with *Plasmodium falciparum* have a lower parasite burden and fewer cerebral complications. It is thought that *P. falciparum*-infected erythrocytes are sequestered in peripheral microvascular beds where oxygen tension is lower and erythrocytes sickle. Although the mechanism is unclear, the replication of the *P. falciparum* is inhibited by sickled cells, thus reducing the severity of the disease.

Related conditions

Mutations in *HBB* that decrease the concentration of β-globin cause β-thalassemia (MIM 141900).

References

Bunn HF. Pathogenesis and treatment of sickle cell disease. N Engl J Med 1997;337:762–9.

Gladwin MT, Rodgers GP. Pathogenesis and treatment of acute chest syndrome of sickle-cell anemia. Lancet 2000;355:1476–8.

Knight J, Murphy TM, Browning I. The lung in sickle cell disease. Pediatr Pulmonol 1999;28:205–16.

Activated Protein C Resistance

(also known as: Factor V Leiden; APC resistance)

MIM 227400

Clinical features Heterozygotes have four to ten times the normal risk of developing a pulmonary embolus or deep venous thrombosis, whereas homozygotes have a 50–100 times greater risk. The frequency of development of pulmonary embolus in patients with deep venous thrombosis is lower in those with activated protein C (APC) resistance than normals, but the absolute number of patients who develop deep venous thrombosis and pulmonary emboli is higher than normals. It does not appear that patients have an increased risk of arterial thrombosis unless they have other risk factors (e.g. smoking, hyperlipidemia).

Age of onset Thromboemboli may begin to occur in adulthood, and the risk increases with age.

Epidemiology Two to twelve percent of European and North American populations, and 20–50% of those with venous thrombosis, are heterozygotes.

Inheritance Autosomal dominant with variable penetrance

Chromosomal location 1q23

Genes *F5* is a 25-exon gene spread over 80 kb that encodes the 2224-amino acid factor V protein. Factor V, a prothrombotic component of the coagulation cascade, is normally cleaved and inactivated by APC.

Mutational spectrum In Factor V Leiden, arginine 506 is replaced by glutamine ($R^{506}Q$). This is the only mutation known to cause APC resistance.

Effect of mutation

Normally, factor V is inactivated by cleavage at position 506, followed by cleavage at position 306. Factor V Leiden, which cannot be cleaved at codon 506, is cleaved only at codon 306, resulting in retention of approximately 10% of normal activity.

Diagnosis

Dilutions of the patient's plasma are mixed with factor V-deficient plasma, and either activated partial thromboplastin time (APTT) or a tissue factor-dependent factor V assay is performed. If activity is low, diagnosis can be confirmed by PCR of genomic DNA, followed by restriction enzyme digestion of the product.

Counselling issues

Pregnancy and oral contraceptive pills markedly increase the risk of venous thromboemboli.

Related conditions

Complete deficiency of factor V has rarely been reported; more common is compound heterozygosity of factor V Leiden with factor V deficiency. These patients are called "pseudohomozygous," because laboratory tests show APC resistance and an APTT in the range of factor V Leiden homozygotes.

References

Bauer KA. Inherited and acquired hypercoagulable states. In: Loscalzo J, Schafer AI, editors. Thrombosis and Hemorrhage. 2nd ed. Baltimore: Williams and Wilkins; 1998. p. 863–97.

Griffin JH, Petaja J. Activated protein C resistance. In: Schafer AI, editor. Molecular mechanisms of hypercoagulable states. Houston, Texas: Landes Bioscience; 1997. p. 101–23.

Antithrombin III Deficiency

(also known as: ATIII deficiency)

MIM	107300
Clinical features	Due to hypercoagulability of blood, patients develop pulmonary emboli, presenting classically with hemoptysis, chest pain, and dyspnea. Thromboemboli may develop in any vein, including the pulmonary, portal, and mesenteric vasculature, with symptoms dependent on the site of thrombosis. Patients may not respond to heparin therapy because its action depends on antithrombin III.
Age of onset	Onset is after puberty, and the risk of thromboemboli increases with age.
Epidemiology	1:250–5000
Inheritance	Autosomal dominant
Chromosomal location	1q23–q25
Genes	The 13.4-kb *AT3* gene, which includes seven exons, encodes the 58-kD antithrombin III, the principal inhibitor of thrombin, a promoter of fibrin formation in the coagulation cascade. Antithrombin III may also inhibit other coagulation factors earlier in the pathway, with the overall effect of preventing thrombus formation.
Mutational spectrum	There are two types of mutations, those that result in a decreased amount of protein (Type I) and those that cause decreased activity (Type II). Most Type I mutations are due to small insertions or deletions, although larger deletions and missense mutations have been reported. All Type II mutations are single-base replacements.
Effect of mutation	Type I mutations result in truncated proteins, abnormal intracellular mRNA or protein processing, or a shortened half-life of the

circulating protein. Type II mutations alter the reactive or heparin-binding sites or cause other conformational changes. Because the critical action of antithrombin III is inhibition of coagulation, quantitative or qualitative defects that alter its ability to inhibit thrombin and other coagulation factors lead to inappropriate coagulation.

Diagnosis

Diagnosis can be made by assaying the heparin cofactor function of antithrombin III. If this test is positive, the concentration of the protein in plasma should be measured, allowing differentiation of Type I and II mutations. Direct sequence analysis of genomic DNA identifies the specific mutation.

Counselling issues

Pregnant patients are at increased risk of miscarriage or stillbirth. Approximately 55% of patients with ATIII deficiency will develop clinically relevant thromboemboli.

Related conditions

Deficiency of heparin cofactor II (MIM 142360), another inhibitor of thrombin, may also be a risk factor for venous thrombosis.

References

Bauer KA. Inherited and acquired hypercoagulable states. In: Loscalzo J, Schafer AI, editors. Thrombosis and Hemorrhage. 2nd ed. Baltimore: Williams and Wilkins; 1998. p. 863–97.

Lane DA, Bayston TA. Molecular basis of antithrombin action and deficiency. In: Schafer AI, editor. Molecular mechanisms of hypercoagulable states. Houston, Texas: Landes Bioscience; 1997. p. 49–77.

Dysfibrinogenemia

MIM

134820; 134830; 134850

Clinical features

Patients are at increased risk of developing pulmonary emboli and deep venous thromboses, but rarely have arterial thrombi. Prothrombin time and activated partial thromboplastin time are usually normal, but thrombin time and reptilase time are prolonged.

Age of onset

Adolescence to adulthood

Epidemiology

Rare, approximately 300 cases reported

Inheritance

Autosomal dominant with variable penetrance

Chromosomal location

4q28

Genes

Fibrinogen is a 340-kD multimeric complex of four Aα, Bβ and γ chains, which are linked by disulfide bridges near their amino termini to form the central E domain. Thrombin cleaves fibrinopeptides A and B from the Aα and Bβ chains, respectively, to produce fibrin chains that can polymerize together to form a clot. Fibrin polymers are later degraded by plasmin.

Mutational spectrum

Mutations in all three fibrinogen chains have been described. Many different replacements of arginine 275 in the γ chain have been found.

Effect of mutation

Because mutations occur in multiple positions throughout the genes, different mechanisms have been postulated to be responsible for the thrombophilia. These include impaired release of fibrinopeptides A and B, abnormal fibrin polymerization, abnormal thrombin-fibrinogen interactions, ineffective calcium binding, disulfide binding to other plasma proteins, and defective plasmin binding.

Diagnosis Patients usually have a prolonged thrombin time, but diagnosis is made definitively by direct sequence analysis of genomic DNA.

Counselling issues Pregnant women are at increased risk of miscarriage, abruptio placentae, and post-partum thrombosis.

Related conditions Although most mutations in fibrinogen never have clinical manifestations, some may result in a bleeding diasthesis due to afibrinogenemia (MIM 202400), and mutations in the α chain can cause familial amyloidosis (MIM 105200).

Defects in the fibrinolytic pathway that can increase the risk of thrombosis may result from mutations in plasminogen (MIM 173350), tissue plasminogen activator (MIM 173370), or plasminogen activator inhibitor (MIM 173360).

References

Haverkate F, Samama M. Familial dysfibrinogenemia and thrombophilia. Report on a study of the SSC subcommittee on fibrinogen. Thromb Haemost 1995;73:151–161.

Mosesson MW. Dysfibrinogenemia and thrombosis. Semin Thromb Haemost 1999;25:311–319.

Hyperhomocysteinemia

(also known as: Homocystinuria)

MIM 603174

Clinical features Patients are at increased risk of developing pulmonary emboli and deep venous thromboses. Spontaneous pneumothorax has been reported rarely. In contrast to many other thrombophilias, hyperhomocysteinemia is associated with an increased risk of atherosclerosis and arterial thrombosis, including coronary, carotid, cerebrovascular, aortic, and peripheral vascular disease. Homozygotes exhibit mental retardation, ectopia lentis, skeletal abnormalities including pectus excavatum or carinatum, and generalized osteoporosis. Heterozygotes have an increased risk of venous and arterial thrombosis without the other abnormalities seen in homozygotes.

Age of onset Childhood

Epidemiology 1:250 000

Inheritance Autosomal recessive

Chromosomal location 21q22.3

Genes *CBS*, a 23-kb gene spanning 23 exons, encodes cystathione β-synthase, an enzyme composed of four identical 63-kD subunits that trans-sulfurates homocysteine to cystathione using serine as a cosubstrate and pyridoxal phosphate (vitamin B6) as a cofactor. Cystathione is then converted to cysteine by γ-cystathionase.

Mutational spectrum Mutations may occur at any site in the gene. The vast majority are missense mutations, with $I^{278}T$ and $G^{307}S$ comprising approximately half of all cases. Many of the mutations show a founder effect in different populations.

Effect of mutation

Known mutations usually alter the binding site for one of the substrates or cofactors or disrupt the quaternary structure of the enzyme, which results in accumulation of homocysteine in the blood. The mechanism by which homocysteine increases the risk of thrombosis is unknown. Homocysteine can damage the vascular endothelium, which may predispose to clotting.

Diagnosis

Concentrations of homocysteine in serum and urine are elevated in homozygotes, and serum levels are elevated or high-normal in heterozygotes. Because the two most common mutations occur in exon 8, SSCP of this exon followed by restriction enzyme digestion can be used as the first step in DNA testing.

Counselling issues

Pregnant women with hyperhomocysteinemia have an increased risk of miscarriage and abruptio placentae. About 50% of patients respond to vitamin B6 replacement. Deficiencies of vitamins B6 and B12 and folate can also result in elevated serum levels of homocysteine.

Related conditions

Mutations of other genes in the homocysteine pathway may result in clinically significant disease. A 677C→T mutation in methylenetetrahydrofolate reductase (MIM 236250) is associated with mild hyperhomocysteinemia. Theoretically, mutations in either methionine synthase (MIM 156570) or methionine synthase reductase (MIM 602568) might cause elevated levels of homocysteine.

References

Guba SC, Fonseca V, Fink LM. Hyperhomocysteinemia and thrombosis. Semin Thromb Hemost 1999;25:291–309.

Rozen R. Genetic modulation of homocysteinemia. Semin Thromb Hemost 2000;26:255–61.

Protein C/Protein S Deficiencies

MIM

176860 Protein C; 176880 Protein S

Clinical features

Patients are predisposed to develop pulmonary emboli and deep venous thromboses. Thromboemboli may also occur in the mesenteric, hepatic, and portal systems, and there is an increased risk of stroke and transient ischemic attacks. Homozygotes develop neonatal purpura fulminans, severe thrombotic episodes, and death in early infancy.

Age of onset

Manifestations in heterozygotes occur in early adulthood, and the risk increases with age. Homozygotes present in infancy.

Epidemiology

Protein C deficiency occurs symptomatically in about 1:16 000 people, but the allele may be present in up to 1:300–500 people. The incidence of Protein S deficiency is not well known, but is estimated to be 1:33 000 people. Each is found in about 8–10% of all hereditary thromboembolic episodes.

Inheritance

Autosomal dominant

Chromosomal location

PROC; 2q13–q14
PROS1; 3p11.1–q11.2

Genes

PROC, an 11.6-kb gene with nine exons, encodes the 40-kD heavy and 22-kD light chains that exist as the disulfide-linked heterodimer Protein C. Protein S, on the other hand, has a single 635-amino acid chain that is encoded by the *PROS1* gene. Protein C, with Protein S as a cofactor, is the primary inhibitor of coagulation via inactivation of factors V and VIII.

Mutational spectrum

There are two types of Protein C deficiency. Type 1 deficiencies result from decreased amounts of protein, most often due to missense and nonsense mutations. Type 2 deficiencies are due exclusively to missense mutations that alter functional activity of the protein. Three types of Protein S deficiency exist. In type 1, missense mutations and small insertions or deletions lead to low levels of protein. Type 2 mutations (most frequently missense) cause low levels of protein with low enzymatic activity. Type 3 is rare, but is characterized purely by altered enzymatic activity, due to one of five missense mutations. In total, more than 100 mutations have been identified in the *PROC* and *PROS1* genes.

Effect of mutation

Quantitative or qualitative defects in Protein C or S result in abnormal regulation of factors V and VIII in the coagulation cascade, shifting the balance toward coagulation and increasing the likelihood of thromboembolic phenomena.

Diagnosis

Direct sequence analysis of genomic DNA can confirm the diagnosis, based initially on plasma levels and activity of Proteins C and S.

Counselling issues

Pregnancy, surgery, trauma, and use of oral contraception increase the risk of thrombosis. Patients are at increased risk of warfarin-induced skin necrosis.

References

Bauer KA. Inherited and acquired hypercoagulable states. In: Loscalzo J, Schafer AI, editors. Thrombosis and Hemorrhage. 2nd ed. Baltimore: Williams and Wilkins; 1998. p. 863–97.

Marlar RA, Hassell KL. Protein C and Protein S deficiencies. In: Schafer AI, editor. Molecular mechanisms of hypercoagulable states. Houston, Texas: Landes Bioscience; 1997. p. 79–100.

Prothrombin Gene Mutation

(also known as: Prothrombin G20210A mutation; Hyperprothrombinemia)

MIM 176930

Clinical features Patients have a propensity to develop pulmonary emboli and other venous thromboses, especially in the portal, mesenteric, and cerebral veins, although the risk is less than that with other thrombophilias, and they may also have an increased risk of coronary artery thrombosis.

Age of onset Onset is in adulthood, and the risk increases with age.

Epidemiology Prevalence of the allele in the population is approximately 1–4%. It is, however, much more frequent among persons of European ancestry, and is the second most common cause of inherited thrombophilia.

Inheritance Autosomal recessive

Chromosomal location 11p11–q12

Genes Prothrombin, a 622-amino acid, 72-kD protein, is encoded by *F2*, a 14-exon gene spread over 21 kb of genomic DNA. Prothrombin, a vitamin K-dependent cofactor, is cleaved by Factor Xa with the assistance of Factor Va to produce thrombin, which converts fibrinogen into fibrin. Thrombin also has a role in platelet aggregation and endothelial cell activation.

Mutational spectrum G20210A is a replacement of guanine for adenosine in the last nucleotide of the 3′ untranslated region and is the only mutation in F2 known to produce a prothrombotic state.

Effect of mutation The mutation results in elevated plasma levels of prothrombin, which is converted to thrombin, causing a hypercoagulable state with increased risk of thrombosis.

Diagnosis

Diagnosis is confirmed by PCR amplification and restriction enzyme digestion of genomic DNA.

Counselling issues

Patients who also carry the Factor V Leiden mutation have an even greater risk of venous thrombosis. Smoking should be avoided and oral contraception should be taken with care as both increase the risk of thrombosis.

References

Nguyen A. Review and management of patients with the prothrombin G20210A polymorphism. Clin Appl Thrombosis/Hemostasis 2000;6:94–9.

Bauer KA. Inherited and acquired hypercoagulable states. In: Loscalzo J, Schafer AI, editors. Thrombosis and Hemorrhage. 2nd ed. Baltimore: Williams and Wilkins; 1998. p. 863–97.

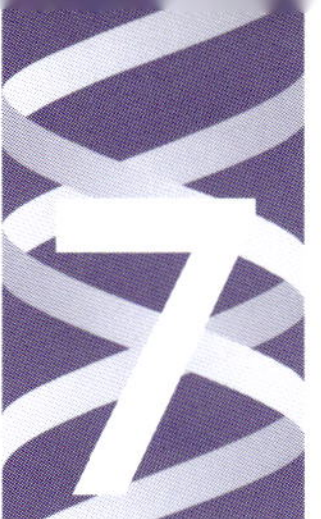

7. Disorders of the pleura/pleural space

Birt-Hogg-Dubé syndrome **110**

Ehlers-Danlos syndrome, vascular type **112**

Familial Mediterranean fever **114**

Marfan's syndrome **117**

TNF receptor-associated periodic syndromes **119**

Birt-Hogg-Dubé Syndrome

(also known as: Fibrofolliculomas with trichodiscomas and acrochordons)

MIM	135150
Clinical features	Patients can develop spontaneous recurrent pneumothoraces due to ruptured lung cysts, but more severe lung disease, including bullous emphysema, can also occur. The principal manifestations of the disease are fibrofolliculomas and trichodiscomas, dome-shaped papules on the head, neck, and upper trunk, and acrochordons, skin tags found on the neck and axilla. Papules may also be present in the oral cavity. Patients have an increased risk of renal neoplasms, and there may be an association with colonic polyps.
Age of onset	Onset occurs after the second decade.
Epidemiology	Rare
Inheritance	Autosomal dominant
Chromosomal location	17p11.2
Genes	Unknown. Because of the cutaneous findings and renal neoplasms, the von Hippel-Landau (VHL) gene was screened, but no mutations were found. Similarly, no mutations were found in the *MET* proto-oncogene, which is associated with papillary renal cell carcinoma.
Mutational spectrum	Unknown
Effect of mutation	It is postulated that the gene, perhaps involved in cell cycle regulation, acts as a tumor suppressor because of its similarities to other diseases with cutaneous and internal organ tumors. The cause of the lung pathology is unknown.
Counselling issues	All patients should be screened for the presence of renal tumors by abdominal CT scan or ultrasound.

Diagnosis Diagnosis is made by histologic examination of dermatologic lesions.

References

Chung JY, Ramos-Caro FA, Beers B, et al. Multiple lipomas, angiolipomas, and parathyroid adenomas in a patient with Birt-Hogg-Dubé syndrome. Int J Dermatol 1996;35:365–7.

Toro JR, Glenn G, Duray P, et al. Birt-Hogg-Dubé syndrome: a novel marker of kidney neoplasia. Arch Dermatol 1999;135:1195–202.

Ehlers-Danlos Syndrome, Vascular Type

(also known as: Ehlers-Danlos syndrome, type IV; Ehlers-Danlos syndrome, arterial type; Ehlers-Danlos Syndrome, ecchymotic type; Ehlers-Danlos syndrome, Sack-Barabas type)

MIM	130050
Clinical features	Pulmonary manifestations include pneumothoraces and pneumohemothoraces. Other features include extensive bruising, rupture of the intestine, uterus, and large arteries, characteristic facies, and thin, translucent skin. Hyperextensibility is usually only present in the digits. The most frequent cause of death is arterial rupture.
Age of onset	Onset is between infancy and late teenage years, but disease may present in early adulthood.
Epidemiology	Rare
Inheritance	Autosomal dominant
Chromosomal location	2q31
Genes	*COL3A1*, spanning 5.5 kb, encodes the 1466-amino acid α-1 chain of type III collagen, which is a primary component of the extracellular matrix in blood vessels, skin, uterus, and gastrointestinal tract. Collagen is composed of three α chains that have repeating amino acid sequences of glycine-x-y wound into a triple helix.
Mutational spectrum	Over 70 mutations are known, most of which cause substitution of glycine for another amino acid. Other mutations cause skipping or deletion of exons, complex splicing patterns with multiple mRNA transcripts, or deletion of single amino acids.
Effect of mutation	Depending on the mutation, there is defective secretion, abnormal posttranslational modification, thermal instability, or sensitivity to

proteases, leading to decreased amounts of α-1-procollagen. A defect in only one of the α chains results in a defective triple helix, so that in a heterozygote only $^1/_8$ ($^1/_2$ x $^1/_2$ x $^1/_2$) of the collagen molecules are normal.

Diagnosis

Diagnosis is made by the presence of abnormal type III procollagen synthesized by fibroblasts cultured from a skin biopsy or by identification of a mutation in the type III collagen gene.

Counselling issues

The first complication is usually noted by age 40 and median age of death is about 50 years old. Pregnancy is associated with increased risk of uterine and arterial rupture, postpartum hemorrhage, and perineal lacerations.

References

Pepin M, Schwarze U, Superti-Furga A, et al. Clinical and genetic features of Ehlers-Danlos syndrome type IV, the vascular type. N Engl J Med 2000;342:673–80.

Pope FM, Burrows NP. Ehlers-Danlos syndrome has varied molecular mechanisms. J Med Genet 1997;34:400–10.

Familial Mediterranean Fever

(also known as: Familial paroxysmal polyserositis; Periodic disease; Recurrent hereditary polyserositis; FMF)

MIM 249100

Clinical features Pleuritis occurs in about one half of patients. Pain is usually unilateral, radiates to the shoulder, and increases with inspiration. Rarely, a pleural friction rub may be heard. There is some evidence of a lower rate of asthma in this population. Fever and sterile peritonitis are the most common manifestations. Monoarticular arthritis of large joints and an erysipelas-like erythema below the knee also occur. Amyloid A (AA) protein amyloidosis, occurring in about 2% of patients, can cause nephrotic syndrome and may progress to renal failure.

Age of onset Childhood to adolescence

Epidemiology The disease is more common in Sephardic Jews (1:5 to 1:16 carriers), Armenians (1:7 carriers), Turks, and Arabs.

Inheritance Autosomal recessive

Chromosomal location 16p13

Genes *MEFV* encodes pyrin/marenostrin, an 86-kD protein of unknown function that is found almost exclusively in granulocytes. It is postulated to be a transcription factor or other effector of nuclear function.

Mutational spectrum Of the 15 identified mutations, $M^{694}V$ is the most common, and several others are found in codons 681–695, indicating that this region is critical for proper protein function. The four most prevalent mutations ($M^{694}V$, $M^{694}I$, $V^{726}A$, and $M^{680}I$) account for 85% of cases.

Effect of mutation

It is not known how the mutation causes the phenotype. One hypothesis is that pyrin/marenostrin is a transcription factor that regulates C5a inhibitor synthesis. In this scenario, subclinical serosal inflammation develops, C5a is activated, and granulocytes are attracted, resulting in a positive feedback loop with unopposed action of inflammatory factors.

Diagnosis

Diagnosis requires the presence of either one major criterion, two minor criteria, one minor criterion and five supportive criteria, or one minor criterion and four of the first five supportive criteria. Major criteria, which must last for 12 hours to 3 days, include peritonitis, unilateral pleuritis, pericarditis, monoarthritis of the knee, ankle, or hip, and fever >38°C. Minor criteria occur during incomplete attacks, are without fever, and involve differing duration of symptoms. They include pain in the abdomen without signs of peritonitis, pain in the chest without pleuritis, arthritis of joints other than the knee, ankle, or hip, exertional leg pain, and positive response to colchicine. Supportive criteria include a positive family history, appropriate ethnic origin, age less than 20 years at disease onset, attacks severe enough to require bedrest, spontaneous remission of attacks, symptom-free intervals, laboratory tests indicative of inflammatory response, episodic proteinuria or hematuria, history of appendectomy with normal histology, and consanguineous parents.

Counselling issues

The disease is most prevalent in Sephardic Jews, Arabs, Armenians, and Turks, but has also been reported in Ashkenazi Jews and Italians. Not all mutations have been identified. Daily 1–2 mg colchicine can be effective in the treatment and prevention of recurrent attacks and amyloidosis.

References

Livneh A, Langevitz P, Pras M. Pulmonary associations in familial Mediterranean fever. Curr Opin Pulm Med 1999;5:326–31.

Samuels J, Aksentijevich I, Torosyan Y, et al. Familial Mediterranean fever at the millennium: clinical spectrum, ancient mutations, and a survey of 100 American referrals to the National Institutes of Health. Medicine 1998;77:268–97.

Booth DR, Gillmore JD, Booth SE, et al. Pyrin/marenostrin mutations in familial Mediterranean fever. QJM 1998;91:603–6

Marfan's Syndrome

(also known as: MFS)

MIM 154700

Clinical features Pneumothorax, most often due to a ruptured apical bleb, is a common manifestation that rarely requires bleb resection and pleurodesis. Pneumothorax occurs more frequently with rapid changes in pressure, such as during scuba diving, ascending an elevator, or riding in an unpressurized airplane. Pulmonary function tests may be spuriously abnormal due to the length of the patients' legs. Usually, there is no pulmonary function test abnormality unless there is severe pectus excavatum or vertebral column deformity. There are various skeletal deformities such as reduced ratio of upper to lower segment, abnormal height, long extremities and digits, and pectus carinatum or excavatum. Other cardinal features include ectopia lentis, dilatation or dissection of the ascending aorta, mitral valve prolapse, and lumbosacral dural ectasia.

Age of onset Congenital

Epidemiology 2–3:10 000

Inheritance Autosomal dominant

Chromosomal location 15q21.1

Genes *FBN1* encodes the 350-kD fibrillin-1 protein that polymerizes to form microfibrils. The gene has 350 exons spanning more than 200 kb. Microfibrils function as scaffolding to distribute stress on the elastin fibers, as anchors for intracellular structures, as bridges between cells and the extracellular matrix, and, possibly, as connectors between epithelial cells and the basement membrane.

Mutational spectrum

Almost all mutations are unique to each family. Over 140 mutations have been identified so far, most of which are missense. Splice-site mutations are also relatively common.

Effect of mutation

It is believed that the mutant allele interferes with the function of the wild-type allele, the so-called dominant negative model. Normally, fibrillin monomers aggregate into microfibrils. A threshold amount of mutant protein prevents appropriate assembly of polymers, creating abnormal microfibrils.

Diagnosis

Clinical diagnosis is based on the presence of major criteria in at least two organ systems (skeletal, ocular, cardiovascular, or skin and integument) and involvement of a third organ system. There are no major pulmonary criteria, but minor criteria are spontaneous pneumothorax or an apical bleb seen on chest X-ray. Family history is highly suggestive if other marfanoid characteristics are present. Molecular diagnosis is rarely made.

Counselling issues

Prenatal diagnosis can be made using amniocytes if the parent's mutation is known. About one quarter of cases are due to new mutations. With proper medical or surgical therapy (β-adrenergic blockers and thoracic aorta surgery), life expectancy is almost normal.

Related conditions

Mutations in FBN1 also cause ectopia lentis (MIM 129600), Shprintzen-Goldberg syndrome (MIM 182212), contractural arachnodactyly (MIM 121050), MASS phenotype (MIM 604308), and familial aortic aneurysm and dissection without classical MFS (MIM 132900).

References

Robinson PN, Godfrey M. The molecular genetics of Marfan syndrome and related microfibrillopathies. J Med Genet 2000;37:9–25.

Pyeritz RE. The Marfan syndrome. Annu Rev Med 2000;51:481–510.

TNF Receptor-Associated Periodic Syndrome

(also known as: TRAPS; Familial Hibernian fever; FHF; Familial periodic fever; FPF)

MIM 142680

Clinical features Attacks of dyspnea and pleuritic chest pain are often due to chest muscle myalgia, pleural effusions, or pleural adhesions. Peak flow rate and chest auscultation are normal. Other characteristics include attacks of fever, abdominal pain and adhesions, erysipelas-like skin lesions, conjunctival injection, periorbital edema, scrotal pain, amyloidosis, and cervical, axillary, and inguinal lymphadenopathy.

Age of onset Infancy to childhood

Epidemiology Rare

Inheritance Autosomal dominant

Chromosomal location 12p13.2

Genes *TNFRSF1A* encodes the 55-kD tumor necrosis factor-α receptor (TNFR1), which upregulates leukocyte adhesion molecules, induces pyrexia, affects responses to intracellular pathogens, increases cytokine secretion, and influences other inflammatory factors. Metalloproteinases cleave membrane-bound TNF-α receptors into a soluble form, which causes a reduction in the downstream activity of the TNF signaling pathway and attenuates the inflammatory response.

Mutational spectrum Of the 14 known mutations, 13 disrupt disulfide bonds by replacing a cysteine or another amino acid near a critical cysteine. The other mutation results in the insertion of four amino acids that alter a region rich in disulfide bonds.

Effect of mutation Impaired shedding of the TNF-α receptor decreases levels of the soluble form and increases levels of the membrane-bound form, leading to increased autoinflammation. Therefore, during times of stress (e.g. infection) when TNF levels are high, inappropriately exuberant inflammatory responses are observed.

Diagnosis

Diagnosis is established by family history, followed by sequence analysis of genomic DNA.

Counselling issues

FHF and FPF were originally designated as separate diseases because FPF patients do not have amyloidosis. However, since the patients with FPF were all from one family with a $C^{52}F$ mutation in *TNFRSF1A*, FHF and FPF are now classified as one disease, TRAPS (TNF-receptor-associated periodic syndromes), to indicate that they are due to mutations in the same gene. Although colchicine can be used as prophylaxis for attacks in Familial Mediterranean Fever (MIM 249100), it is not effective in TRAPS.

References

McDermott EM, Smillie DM, Powell RJ. Clinical spectrum of familial Hibernian fever: a 14-year follow-up study of the index case and extended family. Mayo Clin Proc 1997;72(9):806–17.

McDermott MF, Aksentijevich I, Galon J, et al. Germline mutations in the extracellular domains of the 55 kD TNF receptor, TNFR1, define a family of dominantly inherited autoinflammatory syndromes. Cell 1999;97:133–44.

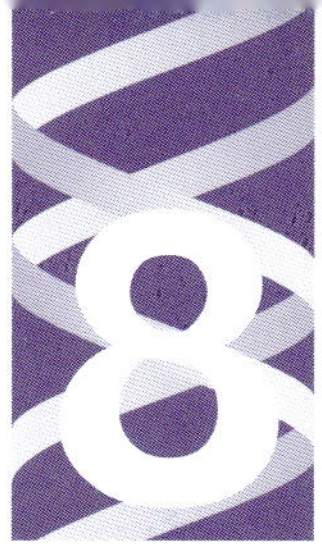

8. Immunodeficiencies

Ataxia-telangiectasia 122

Bloom's syndrome 124

Chronic granulomatous disease 126

Hyper-IgE syndrome 128

Leukocyte mycobactericidal defect 130

Major histocompatibility complex class I deficiency 132

Major histocompatibility complex class II deficiency 134

Severe combined immunodeficiency due to adenosine deaminase deficiency 136

Severe combined immunodeficiency, T-negative, B-positive 138

Severe combined immunodeficiency, T-negative, B-negative 140

Severe combined immunodeficiency due to Zap-70 deficiency 142

Wiskott-Aldrich syndrome 144

X-linked agammaglobulinemia 146

X-linked hyper-IgM syndrome 148

Ataxia-Telangiectasia

(also known as: Louis-Bar syndrome; AT)

MIM	208900
Clinical features	Patients present with recurrent pneumonia and bronchitis, possibly leading to bronchiectasis and pulmonary fibrosis. Pulmonary abscesses, sinusitis, otitis media, pharyngitis, impetigo, skin abscesses, and urinary tract infections have been noted. Gait and truncal ataxia, other neurologic impairments, and oculocutaneous telangiectases are characteristic. Patients have an increased risk of malignancies.
Age of onset	Ataxia is usually noted when the child is learning to walk, and infections are common by the age of 3.
Epidemiology	3:1 000 000
Inheritance	Autosomal recessive
Chromosomal location	11q22.3
Genes	The *ATM* gene, which spans 66 exons, yields a 12-kb transcript encoding a protein involved in mitogenic signal transduction, meiotic signal recombination, cell cycle control, and response to DNA damage. It is one of a family of proteins that all have phosphatidyl inositol 3-kinase-like domains.
Mutational spectrum	70% of the >150 mutations result in either truncation or deletion of a large segment of the protein. Most mutations are specific to each family, although founder effects have been observed in Japanese, Norwegian, and Moroccan-Jewish populations.

Effect of mutation

There is marked sensitivity to ionizing radiation, possibly due to the failure of *ATM* to upregulate p53, which may explain the high incidences of malignancies. Reasons for the immunodeficiency, ataxia, and telangiectases are not known.

Diagnosis

If the family mutation is known, polymerase chain reaction single strand conformational polymorphism (PCR-SSCP) can be performed. Otherwise, the diagnosis is usually made clinically based on ataxia and telangiectases in a child, because so many mutations have been identified.

Counselling issues

Carrier diagnosis may be important because heterozygotes might also have an increased risk of malignancies, especially breast cancer.

Related conditions

Nijmegen Breakage Syndrome (MIM 251260) is a chromosomal instability syndrome in which patients have immunologic and cytogenetic abnormalities and a predisposition to malignancies similar to AT, but without ataxia or telangiectases. Patients also have microcephaly, growth retardation, and abnormalities of sexual and psychomotor development.

References

Lavin MF, Shiloh Y. Ataxia-telangiectasia. In: Ochs HD, Smith CIE, Puck JM, editors. Primary Immunodeficiency Diseases: A Molecular and Genetic Approach. New York: Oxford University Press; 1999. p. 306–23.

McFarlin DE, Strober W, Waldmann TA. Ataxia-telangiectasia. Medicine (Baltimore) 1972;51:281–314.

Bloom's Syndrome

(also known as: BS)

MIM 210900

Clinical features A generalized immunodeficiency predisposes patients to possibly fatal acute pulmonary infections. Chronic pneumonia and bronchitis may lead to bronchiectasis or pulmonary fibrosis. There is an increased risk of malignancies in several organ systems. Men are infertile, and both sexes have a thin face with malar hypoplasia, cardiomyopathy, and dermatologic manifestations that include photosensitivity, telangiectases, and spotty hypo- and hyperpigmented skin.

Age of onset Infancy

Epidemiology Prevalence is 1:10 000 in Ashkenazi Jews, but rare in other populations.

Inheritance Autosomal recessive

Chromosomal location 15q26.1

Genes *BLM*, with a complementary DNA (cDNA) of 4.4 kb, encodes an adenosine triphosphate (ATP)-dependent RecQ family helicase, a 1417-amino acid protein that unwinds double-stranded DNA.

Mutational spectrum The most frequent mutation is a 6-bp deletion (ATCTGA)/7-bp insertion (TAGATTC) at nucleotide 2281 of the *BLM* cDNA, known as blm(ASH). Others include missense, deletion, and insertion mutations.

Effect of mutation Most mutations result in an inability of the protein to unwind DNA due to disruption of the DNA-binding domain or interference with ATPase activity. In addition, the abnormal BLM gene product may disturb the function of other enzymes involved in DNA repair and replication (e.g. topoisomerases and ligases).

Diagnosis

A PCR-based test has been developed for the Ashkenazi Jewish mutation that can be used to screen homozygotes or carriers of the mutant allele.

Counselling issues

Patients usually die in their teens or early adulthood.

References

Rong SB, Valiaho J, Vihinen M. Structural basis of Bloom Syndrome (BS) causing mutations in the BLM helicase domain. Mol Med 2000;6:155–64.

German J, Passarge E. Bloom's Syndrome. XII. Report from the Registry for 1987. Clin Genet 1989;35:57–69.

Chronic Granulomatous Disease

(also known as: CGD)

MIM

306400; 233690; 233700; 233710

Clinical features

Pneumonia is the most frequent infection with over one third of cases due to the fungus *Aspergillus*. *Staphylococcus*, *Burkholderia*, *Nocardia*, *Serratia*, and *Mycobacteria* are other known causative agents. These organisms may cause abscesses in the lung, as well as in the skin, liver, brain, and perirectal area. Patients also develop suppurative adenitis, osteomyelitis, bacteremia, cellulitis, and meningitis. Other noninfectious disorders include lupus syndromes, gastric or urinary outlet obstruction, colitis, idiopathic thrombocytopenic purpura, and chorioretinitis.

Age of onset

Onset is usually in childhood, but may occur later in autosomal recessive cases.

Epidemiology

The prevalence is 1:200 000, but because the most common form is X-linked most patients are males.

Inheritance

X-linked recessive (MIM 306400); autosomal recessive (MIM 233690, 233700, 233710)

Chromosomal location

CYBB; Xp21.1
CYBA; 16q24
NCF1; 7q11.23
NCF2; 1q25

Genes

All the genes encode for components of the NADPH oxidase complex. *CYBB*, the gene for the gp91*phox* component, spans 13 exons on the X-chromosome and encodes a 570-amino acid protein. The three autosomal recessive genes are: *CYBA*, encoding the p22*phox* component on chromosome 16; *NCF1*, encoding the p47*phox* component on chromosome 7; and *NCF2*, encoding the p67*phox* component on chromosome 1.

Mutational spectrum

Most of the reported frameshift, nonsense, and missense mutations in *CYBB* are family-specific. Many fewer mutations have been reported in the autosomal genes, but missense mutations are most common in *CYBA*. A two-nucleotide deletion is by far the most frequent mutation in *NCF1*, and various frameshift deletions are common in *NCF2*.

Effect of mutation

The mutations render the NADPH oxidase system unable to produce superoxide anion or other toxic oxygen metabolites. Therefore, although phagocytosis of pathogens is not impaired, leukocytes are defective in intracellular destruction of the infective agents.

Diagnosis

Diagnosis is made by sequence analysis of exons that show abnormal migration patterns on SSCP screening.

Counselling issues

The X-linked form has been documented in women who have skewed lyonization of the X-chromosome. Patients with the X-linked form usually live into their third decade, whereas patients with the autosomal recessive forms live into their fifth decade. Interferon-γ and prophylactic trimethoprim-sulfamethoxazole reduce the incidence of infections.

References

Segal BH, Leto TL, Gallin JI, et al. Genetic, biochemical, and clinical features of chronic granulomatous disease. Medicine (Baltimore) 2000;79:170–200.

Winkelstein JA, Marino MC, Johnston RB Jr, et al. Chronic granulomatous disease. Report on a national registry of 368 patients. Medicine (Baltimore) 2000;79:155–69.

Hyper-IgE Syndrome

(also known as: Job syndrome; Hyper-IgE recurrent infection syndrome)

MIM	147060; 243700
Clinical features	Pneumonia is most often due to *Haemophilus influenzae*, *Staphylococcus aureus*, and *Pneumocystis carinii*. Pneumatoceles may become superinfected with *Pseudomonas aeruginosa* or *Aspergillus fumigatus*. Bronchiectasis may develop after repeated infections. Retained primary teeth, distinctive facies, multiple bone fractures, scoliosis, eczema, candidiasis, abscesses, osteomyelitis, lymphoma, and joint hyperextensibility have also been noted. Characteristic laboratory results include eosinophilia and elevated IgE.
Age of onset	Childhood
Epidemiology	Rare
Inheritance	Autosomal dominant with variable expressivity
Chromosomal location	4q21
Genes	Unknown
Mutational spectrum	A founder effect is unlikely because patients have varied ethnic backgrounds and, in the past, most did not live to reproductive age.
Effect of mutation	Mutations result in abnormalities of the immune, skeletal, and connective-tissue systems, but the underlying defect is unknown.
Diagnosis	Diagnosis is based on the combination of elevated serum IgE concentrations, eczematoid rashes, and unusual, recurrent infections such as skin abscesses, candidiasis, and pneumonias with pneumatocele formation.

Counselling issues

Aggressive antibiotic treatment should be instituted for infections, and surgical drainage may be necessary for pneumatoceles and abscesses. Full evaluations should be performed for fractures after minor trauma. Retained primary teeth should be removed.

References

Grimbacher B, Schaffer AA, Holland SM, et al. Genetic linkage of hyper-IgE syndrome to chromosome 4. Am J Hum Genet 1999;65:735–44.

Grimbacher B, Holland SM, Gallin JI, et al. Hyper-IgE syndrome with recurrent infections – an autosomal dominant multisystem disorder. N Engl J Med 1999;340:692–702.

Leukocyte Mycobactericidal Defect

(also known as: Familial atypical mycobacteriosis)

MIM
209950

Clinical features
Disseminated infection with atypical mycobacteria or Bacillus Calmette-Guerin (BCG) characteristically affects the lungs and lymph nodes, which may lead to bronchial obstruction or lung consolidation. Histologically, failure to form mature granulomas is seen. Prevalence of asthma and atopy is high. Mycobacteria can infiltrate viscera, blood, and bone marrow. Other signs include fever, hepatosplenomegaly, lymphadenopathy, positive paired-pulse depression (PPD), and chronic anemia. Frequency of *Salmonella*, *Listeria*, *Mycoplasma pneumoniae*, and herpes virus infections is also increased.

Age of onset
Infancy

Epidemiology
Rare

Inheritance
Autosomal recessive

Chromosomal location
IFNGR1; 6q23–q24
IFNGR2; 21q22.1–q22.2
IL12RB1; 19p13.1
IL12B; 5q31.1–q33.1

Genes
Mutations have been identified in several components of the IFN-γ and IL-12 pathways: the IFN-γ receptor-1 gene, *IFNGR1*, on chromosome 6; the IFN-γ receptor-2 gene, *IFNGR2*, on chromosome 21; the β1 chain of the IL-12 receptor, *IL12RB1*, on chromosome 19; and the 45-kD chain of IL-12, *IL12B*, on chromosome 5.

Mutational spectrum

Complete deficiencies of the various proteins are due to insertion, deletion, or nonsense mutations that result in truncated proteins. One missense and one splice-site mutation in *IFNGR1* and one missense mutation in *IFNGR2* have also been reported.

Effect of mutation

IL-12 induces IFN-γ production by T cells and natural killer cells. IFN-γ activates numerous genes involved in immune functions, including antigen processing and presentation, apoptosis, and production of TNF-α. IFN-γ also causes destruction of mycobacteria through a poorly defined mechanism.

Diagnosis

Direct sequence analysis of genomic DNA is confirmatory.

Counselling issues

Antibiotics will not completely eradicate the pathogens and patients remain susceptible to further mycobacterial infections. Bone marrow transplantation may eliminate susceptibility in patients with mutations in *IFNGR1*. Because live mycobacterial vaccines may result in infection, BCG vaccine should not be given to these patients.

Related conditions

Autosomal dominant IFNGR1 deficiency has been reported in various kindreds, almost always due to a specific frameshift deletion. Administration of exogenous IFN-γ can reduce disease severity.

References

Dorman SE, Holland SM. Interferon-γ and interleukin-12 pathway defects and human disease. Cytokine Growth Factor Rev 2000;11:321–33.

Levin M, Newport MJ, D'Souza S, et al. Familial disseminated atypical mycobacterial infection in childhood: a human mycobacterial susceptibility gene? Lancet 1995;345:79–83.

Major Histocompatibility Complex Class I Deficiency

(also known as: MHCI deficiency; Bare lymphocyte syndrome, type I; BLS, type I; TAP deficiency syndrome)

MIM 604571

Clinical features Purulent rhinitis, nasal polyposis and septal perforation, sinusitis, otitis media, and post-nasal drip are early manifestations. Later, pneumonia and spastic bronchitis due to *Haemophilus influenza, Streptococcus pneumoniae, Staphylococcus aureus, Klebsiella, Escherichia coli,* and *Pseudomonas aeruginosa* are common. Susceptibility to viral pathogens is not increased. By late childhood, chronic lung disease including bronchiectasis, panbronchiolitis, emphysema, and bronchial obstruction occur. Necrotizing granulomatous skin lesions, vasculitis, and cerebral abscesses have been noted. Chronic diarrhea and systemic infections are not seen in these patients. Cells have low or absent MHC class I expression, and patients have a deficiency of CD8+, but not CD4+, cells.

Age of onset Infections begin by late childhood.

Epidemiology Ten patients are known worldwide.

Inheritance Autosomal recessive

Chromosomal location 6p21.3

Genes *TAP1* and *TAP2*, which encode the 808- and 653-amino acid subunits of TAP (transporter associated with antigen processing), respectively, reside in the Class II HLA locus on chromosome 6. TAP chaperones peptide antigens from the cytosol through the Golgi apparatus to the endoplasmic reticulum where they complex with MHC I molecules before transport to the cell surface.

Mutational spectrum

Two mutations have been identified in *TAP1*, a splice-site mutation at exon 2 and a single base-pair deletion at position 819, and two in *TAP2*, a nonsense mutation at codon 273 and a single base-pair deletion in codon 326.

Effect of mutation

In TAP deficiency antigens are not delivered to the endoplasmic reticulum and MHC I molecules are degraded intracellularly. It is thought that lung damage is initiated by subacute viral infection, which causes loss of cilia and fibrosis, predisposing to chronic bacterial colonization.

Diagnosis

Absence of MHC I molecules detected by flow cytometry is diagnostic.

Counselling issues

As in cystic fibrosis, chronic lung infection should be managed with appropriate antibiotics and chest physiotherapy. Patients should be counselled to avoid smoking.

Related conditions

One completely asymptomatic family without MHC I expression has been reported. In addition, a more severe phenotype with infections earlier in life has been described, but a genetic locus has not been found.

References

de la Salle H, Donato L, Zimmer J, et al. HLA Class I deficiencies. In: Ochs HD, Smith CIE, Puck JM, editors. Primary Immunodeficiency Diseases: A Molecular and Genetic Approach. New York: Oxford University Press; 1999. p. 181–8.

Gadola SD, Moins-Teisserenc HT, Trowsdale J, et al. TAP deficiency syndrome. Clin Exp Immunol 2000;121:173–8.

Major Histocompatibility Complex Class II deficiency

(also known as: MHC II deficiency; Type II Bare Lymphocyte Syndrome; Type II BLS)

MIM 209920

Clinical features Almost all patients develop repeated episodes of pneumonia and bronchitis. *Pseudomonas, Streptococcus, Haemophilus, Staphylococcus, Proteus, Pneumocystis carinii, Candida albicans,* cytomegalovirus (CMV), respiratory syncytial virus, and enterovirus are reported etiologic agents. Chronic infectious diarrhea, including colonization by *Cryptosporidium*, can lead to malnutrition or failure to thrive. Hepatitis, cholangitis, meningoencephalitis, chronic lymphocytic meningitis, and poliomyelitis have been observed. The characteristic laboratory finding is absence of MHC II on B cells and phytohemagglutinin (PHA)-activated T cells. Serum immunoglobulin levels may be low or normal, but there is usually a negative response to immunizations and microbial antigens. Delayed-type hypersensitivity is completely absent.

Age of onset Onset is within the first year.

Epidemiology Prevalence is rare with only 70 patients from 57 families, mostly from North Africa, reported.

Inheritance Autosomal recessive

Chromosomal location *MHC2TA;* 16p13
RFXANK; 19p12
RFX5; 1q21.1–q21.3
RFXAP; 13q14

Genes Four genes have been found to cause this disease: MHC2TA on chromosome 16, RFXANK on chromosome 19, RFX5 on chromosome 1, and RFXAP on chromosome 13. These genes control the regulation of expression of the MHC II genes. MHC II presents antigens to T cell receptors on CD4+ cells to activate antigen-specific T cells.

Mutational spectrum

Two large deletions and a nonsense mutation have been identified in *MHC2TA*. Mutations in *RFXANK* include two small deletions, a nonsense mutation, and a missense mutation. Five known mutations in *RFX5* include two nonsense and three splice-site mutations. Lastly, four small insertions and one nonsense mutation have been found in *RFXAP*.

Effect of mutations

Lack of expression of MHC II on professional antigen-presenting cells (e.g. B cells, skin Langerhans cells, and hepatic Kupffer cells) results in an abnormal immune response to virulent organisms.

Diagnosis

Laboratory tests confirm absence of MHC II and of antibody response to specific immunization antigens. Sequence analysis of genomic DNA can then identify the affected gene.

Counselling issues

HLA-matched bone marrow transplantation should be attempted as soon as possible after diagnosis. Untreated patients usually die between ages 5 and 14. Live, attenuated vaccines should not be given.

References

DeSandro A, Nagarajan UM, Boss JM. The bare lymphocyte syndrome: molecular clues to the transcriptional regulation of major histocompatibility complex class II genes. Am J Hum Genet 1999;65:279–86.

Reith W, Steimle V, Lisowska-Grospierre B, et al. Molecular basis of major histocompatibility complex class II deficiency. In: Ochs HD, Smith CIE, Puck JM, editors. Primary Immunodeficiency Diseases: A Molecular and Genetic Approach. New York: Oxford University Press; 1999. p. 167–80.

Severe Combined Immunodeficiency due to Adenosine Deaminase Deficiency

(also known as: ADA-SCID)

MIM 102700

Clinical features The presenting manifestations are often pneumonia, bronchitis, and bronchiolitis due to opportunistic pathogens, including respiratory syncytial virus, *Pneumocystis carinii*, and parainfluenza type 3. Chronic lung damage and severe alveolitis requiring mechanical ventilation have been reported in the adult-onset form. Oral, gluteal, and vaginal candidiasis, sinusitis, adenovirus infection, disseminated varicella, and Gram-negative sepsis are also common. Chronic diarrhea, hepatosplenomegaly, and failure to thrive are often noted. Profound lymphocytopenia involving B-, T-, and natural killer cells, hypogammaglobulinemia, thymic atrophy, and absence of delayed-type hypersensitivity are characteristic abnormalities. Graft-versus-host disease occurs in a significant proportion of patients due to placental transfer of maternal lymphocytes. Cupping and flaring of rib ends may be seen on chest X-ray.

Age of onset Most patients present in the first year. About 20%, however, have a less severe course and are diagnosed later in childhood or in early adulthood.

Epidemiology The prevalence is 1–5:1 000 000, which is about 15% of all cases of SCID.

Inheritance Autosomal recessive

Chromosomal location 20q13.11

Genes *ADA* is a 12-exon gene that encodes adenosine deaminase, a 41-kD protein that functions in the purine salvage pathway and converts adenosine and 2′-deoxyadenosine to inosine or 2′-deoxyinosine, respectively.

Mutational spectrum Almost all patients are heteroallelic, having different mutations on each allele. Most of the over 50 mutations are within a part of the gene distant from the adenosine deaminase (ADA) catalytic site.

Effect of mutation The absence of ADA causes a buildup of lymphotoxic precursors, specifically deoxyadenosine. Elevated levels of deoxyadenosine inhibit ribonucleotide reductase, killing nondividing cells through the accumulation of DNA-strand breaks, and inducing apoptosis through the p53 and caspase pathways. In addition, deoxyadenosine inhibits the activity of S-adenosylhomocysteine hydrolase with resultant decrease in S-adenosylmethionine-dependent methylation reactions and possible induction of apoptosis through a Fas-mediated mechanism.

Diagnosis ADA levels may be quantified in hemolysates. Elevated levels of erythrocyte deoxyadenosine triphosphate (dATP) are diagnostic. Disease may be confirmed by sequence analysis of genomic DNA.

Counselling issues ADA deficiency is fatal in the first year of life without HLA-matched bone marrow transplantation. An alternative therapy is PEG-ADA, adenosine deaminase modified with attachment of polyethylene glycol. Prenatal diagnosis can be made using chorionic villus sampling.

Related conditions Deficiency of purine nucleoside phosphorylase (MIM 164050), the enzyme after ADA in the degradation pathway, has a phenotype similar to ADA deficiency, except for more severe T cell dysfunction.

References

Buckley RH, Schiff RI, Schiff SE, et al. Human severe combined immunodeficiency: genetic, phenotypic, and functional diversity in 108 infants. J Pediatr 1997;130:378–87.

Hershfield MS. Adenosine deaminase deficiency: clinical expression, molecular basis, and therapy. Semin Hematol 1998;35:291–8.

Severe Combined Immunodeficiency, T-negative, B-positive

(also known as: SCID; Swiss type agammaglobulinemia; Thymic epithelial hypoplasia; Immunodeficiency 4)

MIM

300400; 600173

Clinical features

Presentation is often pneumonia due to respiratory syncytial virus, parainfluenza type 3, CMV, *Candida* and other fungi, *Pneumocystis carinii*, and *Pseudomonas*. Other manifestations include oral and gluteal candidiasis, chronic diarrhea, bacterial meningitis, failure to thrive, and gram-negative sepsis. Lymphocytopenia, agammaglobulinemia, decrease in the number of natural killer cells, absence of delayed-type hypersensitivity, absent tonsils, and thymic atrophy are characteristic immunologic abnormalities. Graft-versus-host disease may occur due to transplacentally-derived maternal lymphocytes.

Age of onset

Within the first year

Epidemiology

1:50 000–500 000

Inheritance

X-linked recessive (MIM 300400); autosomal recessive (MIM 600173)

Chromosomal location

IL2RG; Xq13
JAK3; 19p13.1

Genes

The *IL2RG* gene, encoding the interleukin-2 receptor γ chain, is a subunit of the IL-2, IL-4, IL-7, IL-9, and IL-15 receptors. Each receptor is composed of the γ chain and one or two noncovalently linked, receptor-specific chains. *IL2RG* has eight exons, encoding a 369-amino acid, 65-kD protein.

The *JAK3* gene encodes Janus kinase 3, with an mRNA of 4604 nucleotides and a protein product of 1124 amino acids. The carboxy-terminus of the shared interleukin receptor γ chain associates with *JAK3* to initiate signaling in the interleukin pathway.

Mutational spectrum

About 150 mutations have been identified in *IL2RG*; most frequent are missense and nonsense mutations in exons 3, 4, and 5. There is a high frequency of mutations of nucleotides 661–691, with $R^{222}C$, $R^{224}W$, $R^{226}C$, and $R^{226}H$ occurring commonly. Premature terminations at R289 have also been found in several different persons.

Only a few mutations, most commonly nonsense, are known in *JAK3*.

Effect of mutations

The diversity of defects is due to the several interleukin pathways that are impaired. Abnormalities in the IL-7 pathway significantly reduce T cell differentiation. T cells that are present cannot proliferate effectively because of a deficient response to IL-2. The defective IL-4 receptor causes difficulty in B cell Ig class-switching.

Diagnosis

Diagnosis is made by sequence analysis of genomic DNA.

Counselling issues

This diagnosis is a pediatric emergency. If left untreated, death usually occurs from overwhelming infection by 2 years. Bone marrow transplantation as soon as diagnosis is recognized can be curative. Absence of T-lymphocytes from umbilical cord blood can establish prenatal diagnosis.

References

Buckley RH, Schiff RI, Schiff SE, et al. Human severe combined immunodeficiency: genetic, phenotypic, and functional diversity in 108 infants. J Pediatr 1997;130:378–87.

Puck JM. IL2RGbase: a database of γ c-chain defects causing human X-SCID. Immunol Today 1996;17:507–11.

Uribe L, Weinberg KI. X-linked SCID and other defects of cytokine pathways. Semin Hematol 1998;35:299–309.

Severe Combined Immunodeficiency, T-negative, B-negative

(also known as: SCID; Recombination-activating gene (RAG)1 and RAG2 deficiency; Omenn syndrome)

MIM	179615 RAG1; 179616 RAG2; 603554 Omenn syndrome
Clinical features	A defective immune system allows opportunistic pathogens such as *Pneumocystis carinii*, parainfluenza type 3, CMV, adenovirus, fungi, and *Pseudomonas* to cause chronic, recurrent pneumonia, bronchitis, and sinusitis. Oral and gluteal candidiasis, otitis, mastoiditis, rhinitis, conjunctivitis, chronic diarrhea, abscesses, and life-threatening meningitis and sepsis are other infectious complications. In addition, recombination-activating gene (RAG) 1 and RAG2 deficiency are characterized by T cell and B cell lymphocytopenia, normal natural killer cells, absence of cervical lymph nodes and tonsils, and agammaglobulinemia. Omenn syndrome, a less severe form of RAG1 or RAG2 deficiency, is manifested by graft-versus-host disease-like findings, hypereosinophilia, exudative erythrodermia, hepatosplenomegaly, lymphadenopathy, and elevated serum IgE.
Age of onset	Within months of birth
Epidemiology	Less than 1:100 000
Inheritance	Autosomal recessive
Chromosomal location	11p13
Genes	*RAG1* and *RAG2*, located in the same region on chromosome 11, encode 119-kD and 58-kD proteins, respectively, which localize to the nucleus and participate in V(D)J recombination of immunoglobulin and T cell receptors.

Mutational spectrum

The only mutations reported in *RAG1* are three nonsense and two missense mutations. The three mutations found in *RAG2* are $C^{478}Y$, $R^{229}G$, and a 3-bp in-frame deletion resulting in absence of isoleucine 273. Omenn syndrome is known to result from seven missense and two deletion mutations in *RAG1* and three missense mutations in *RAG2*.

Effect of mutation

B cell and T cell differentiation is dependent on immunoglobulin and T cell receptor rearrangements, respectively. When these pathways are affected, pre-B and pre-T cells undergo apoptosis because of failure to receive a survival signal to continue differentiation, which results in an immunodeficient state. In Omenn syndrome, RAG1 or RAG2 retains partial recombinatory activity, and production of some lymphocytes is possible.

Diagnosis

SSCP or direct sequence analysis of genomic DNA provides the diagnosis.

Counselling issues

HLA-matched bone marrow transplantation is required as soon as possible after diagnosis to avoid fatal infections or malnutrition. Vaccines with live, attenuated organisms should be avoided.

Related conditions

Another type of SCID has been found in Athabaskan-speaking Native Americans (MIM 602450), which also seems to be due to V(D)J recombination defects, with the responsible gene localized to chromosome 10p. The disease has a reported incidence of 1:2000 in Navajo Indians. Reticular dysgenesia (MIM 267500) is one of the most rare and fatal forms of SCID. No chromosomal location or gene product has been identified.

References

Schwarz K, Notarangelo LD, Spanopoulou E, et al. Recombination Defects. In: Ochs HD, Smith CIE, Puck JM, editors. Primary Immunodeficiency Diseases: A Molecular and Genetic Approach. New York: Oxford University Press; 1999. p. 155–66.

Villa A, Santagata S, Bozzi F, et al. Omenn syndrome: a disorder of Rag1 and Rag2 genes. J Clin Immunol 1999;19:87–97.

Severe Combined Immunodeficiency due to Zap-70 Deficiency

(also known as: CD8 Lymphopenia)

MIM 176947

Clinical features *Pneumocystis carinii* pneumonia and parainfluenza pneumonitis may be the presenting signs. Other infectious complications include otitis media, CMV retinitis, chronic diarrhea from rotavirus or other agents, disseminated varicella, and oral candidiasis. Failure to thrive is also a common sign. A thymic shadow is seen on chest X-ray. Deficiency of CD8+ T cells with a compensatory increased percentage of CD4+ cells is observed. B cells are normal in number and function.

Age of onset Onset is within the first 2 years.

Epidemiology Eight patients in five families have been reported.

Inheritance Autosomal recessive

Chromosomal location 2q12

Genes The T cell receptor ζ-chain-associated protein kinase, encoded by the gene *ZAP70*, is a 70-kD member of the protein tyrosine kinase family. When a ligand binds the T cell receptor, ZAP70 is phosphorylated and associates with various SH2 domain-containing proteins, allowing for downstream signaling in T cells.

Mutational spectrum Three known mutations are a replacement of guanine by adenine with a 9-bp deletion after nucleotide 1832; an $S^{518}R$ missense mutation; and a 13-bp deletion (nucleotides 1719–1731) resulting in a frameshift and termination. One patient was found to have no ZAP70 mRNA, but the mutation has not been identified.

Effect of mutation

All the mutations affect the stability of the protein and/or alter the catalytic region. One theory holds that ZAP70 is necessary for T-lymphocyte differentiation. CD4+, but not CD8+, cells are able to compensate for the loss of ZAP70 by upregulation of Syk, another protein kinase in the pathway.

Diagnosis

Genomic sequencing is the current diagnostic method.

Counselling issues

HLA-matched bone marrow transplantation is the accepted therapy and should be instituted as soon as possible to avoid infectious complications.

Related conditions

A defect in p56lck (MIM 153390), another protein tyrosine kinase that is involved in T cell receptor signaling, was found in one child who presented with failure to thrive, sepsis, rotaviral diarrhea, and CMV in the urine and intestinal biopsy. He was later found to have CD4+ lymphopenia but normal numbers of CD8+ cells. Deficiencies have also been noted in CD3ϵ (MIM 186830) and CD3γ (MIM 186740) that result in decreased numbers of CD3+ and CD4+ T cells, but normal CD8+ and B-lymphocytes. These patients have abnormal T cell receptor signaling and, therefore, are prone to opportunistic infections.

References

Elder ME. ZAP-70 and defects of T cell receptor signaling. Semin Hematol 1998;35:310–20.

Elder ME, Weiss A. SCID resulting from mutations in the gene encoding the protein tyrosine kinase ZAP-70. In: Ochs HD, Smith CIE, Puck JM, editors. Primary Immunodeficiency Diseases: A Molecular and Genetic Approach. New York: Oxford University Press; 1999. p. 146–54.

Wiskott-Aldrich Syndrome

(also known as: Aldrich syndrome)

MIM	301000
Clinical features	Recurrent pneumonia, occasionally due to *Pneumocystis carinii,* is often the first manifestation. Infectious complications include otitis media, sinusitis, chronic diarrhea, impetigo, cellulitis, skin abscesses, sepsis, meningitis, recurrent herpes simplex infections, and candidiasis. Lymphoreticular malignancies occur in late childhood. Thrombocytopenia with purpura, petechiae, epistaxis, hematemesis, and melena are seen. Other hematologic findings include low numbers of T cells, autoimmune hemolytic anemia, elevated amounts of IgA and IgE, and low IgM, but there is wide variation in laboratory values. Absence of delayed-type hypersensitivity and eczema are also common.
Age of onset	Early childhood
Epidemiology	1–4:1 000 000
Inheritance	X-linked recessive
Chromosomal location	Xp11.23–p11.22
Genes	The gene responsible, *WASP*, spans about 9 kb and contains 12 exons. The WASP protein, which has a high content of glycine, leucine, and proline, is present in all cells derived from hematopoietic stem cells and is involved in cytoskeletal reorganization in T cells and platelets.
Mutational spectrum	Over 200 mutations have been reported throughout the entire gene. Most are missense or nonsense, with a high percentage of missense mutations in exons 2 and 4.

Effect of mutation

It is thought that mutations in *WASP* result in defective reorganization of the T cell cytoskeleton upon activation, which interferes with the ability of T cells to interact with B cells and results in an immunodeficient state. In addition, the inability of platelets to alter the cytoskeleton and form filopodia when activated results in platelet destruction and thrombocytopenia.

Diagnosis

SSCP, followed by sequencing of exons with aberrant electrophoretic patterns, can establish the diagnosis.

Counselling issues

Amniocentesis or chorionic villus biopsy can be used for prenatal testing. Cesarean section may reduce trauma to the neonate. Aggressive antibiotic treatment should be instituted if infection is suspected. Intravenous immunoglobulin and bone marrow transplantation have significantly decreased mortality rate. Life expectancy is now about 11 years but many patients live into the third decade.

Related conditions

Autosomal recessive (MIM 277970) and autosomal dominant (MIM 600903) forms have been postulated, but molecular defects have not been identified. Unequal lyonization of the X-chromosome may be responsible for expression of the disease phenotype in females.

References

Ochs HD, Rosen FS. The Wiskott-Aldrich Syndrome. In: Ochs HD, Smith CIE, Puck JM, editors. Primary Immunodeficiency Diseases. New York: Oxford University Press; 1999. p. 292–305.

Sullivan KE, Mullen CA, Blaese RM, et al. A multiinstitutional survey of the Wiskott-Aldrich syndrome. J Pediatr 1994;125:876–85.

X-linked Agammaglobulinemia

(also known as: Bruton type agammaglobulinemia; Immunodeficiency 1)

MIM

300300

Clinical features

Recurrent pneumonia, bronchitis, or bronchiolitis are the presenting signs in many patients. Organisms include *Haemophilus influenza*, *Staphylococcus aureus*, *Streptococcus pneumoniae*, and *Pneumocystis carinii*, but often infections are due to multiple agents. Bronchiectasis and pulmonary fibrosis with cor pulmonale may occur as a complication of infections. Other infections include pyogenic mono- or oligo-articular arthritis of large joints, meningitis, encephalitis, otitis media, sinusitis, chronic diarrhea, pyoderma, and sepsis. Enteroviruses frequently cause chronic meningitis and dermatomyositis. There is characteristically a lack of serum immunoglobulins and a greatly reduced number of B cells.

Age of onset

Onset is within the first year of life, but diagnosis may not be made until adolescence.

Epidemiology

1:200 000

Inheritance

X-linked recessive

Chromosomal location

Xq21.3–q22

Genes

The *BTK* gene, which encodes Bruton tyrosine kinase, contains 19 exons spanning 37 kb with a protein product of 659 amino acids. BTK, a member of the Tec family of protein kinases, is a component of various B cell receptor signaling pathways.

Mutational spectrum

About 400 mutations have been identified, with most in exons 2, 15, and 18. Missense and frameshift deletion mutations are most common.

Effect of mutation

Mutations in BTK cause abnormal B cell signaling, but the mechanism has not been elucidated. B cell differentiation is blocked at the pre-B cell state. These immature precursors cannot produce immunoglobulins, causing a generalized immunodeficiency.

Diagnosis

Laboratory testing reveals low concentrations of all immunoglobulins and lack of antibody response upon antigen challenge. SSCP of genomic DNA followed by sequence analysis should identify the mutation.

Counselling issues

Intravenous immunoglobulin can reduce the frequency of pneumonia and hospitalization, especially when given before the age of 5. Aggressive antibiotic treatment should be instituted if infection is suspected, but, even with proper treatment, the organism might never be fully eradicated. Most patients live well into adulthood.

Related conditions

Two autosomal recessive forms of agammaglobulinemia are due to deficiency of the μ heavy chain on chromosome 14 (MIM 601495) and mutations in the λ5/14.1 gene on chromosome 22 (MIM 146770). It is probable that there are additional genes.

References

Hermaszewski RA, Webster AD. Primary hypogammaglobulinaemia: a survey of clinical manifestations and complications. Q J Med 1993;86:31–42.

Smith CIE, Witte ON. X-linked agammaglobulinemia: a disease of Btk tyrosine kinase. In: Ochs HD, Smith CIE, Puck JM, editors. Primary Immunodeficiency Diseases. New York: Oxford University Press; 1999. p. 263–84.

X-linked Hyper-IgM Syndrome

(also known as: Immunodeficiency 3; Dysgammaglobulinemia type 1)

MIM

308230

Clinical features

Pneumonia due to *Pneumocystis carinii* is the most common presenting sign, but infections with bacteria, CMV, and adenovirus have been reported. *Cryptococcus neoforms* and atypical mycobacteria may be found in the lung. Bronchiectasis develops in one quarter of patients who have lower respiratory tract infections. Patients may also develop severe diarrhea, oral ulcers, sclerosing cholangitis, hepatitis, sepsis, and meningoencephalitis. Hematologic manifestations include elevated or normal IgM, low IgG, IgA, and IgE, normal T and B cell lymphocyte levels, anemia, and neutropenia.

Age of onset

Early childhood

Epidemiology

Less than 1:1 000 000

Inheritance

X-linked recessive

Chromosomal location

Xq26

Genes

CD40LG, which encodes the CD40 ligand, is a member of the tumor necrosis factor (TNF) superfamily. It has five exons, encoding a 39-kD protein that is expressed preferentially on T cells. Interaction of the CD40 ligand with CD40 stimulates immunoglobulin synthesis and B cell proliferation.

Mutational spectrum

Over 70 mutations have been identified in almost 90 families. Most are in exon 5, which encodes the TNF-α homology domain.

Effect of mutation

Defective interaction between CD40 and its ligand results in abnormal B cell differentiation, abnormal immunoglobulin isotype switching, and lack of memory response. CD40 ligand may also be involved in immunity to opportunistic infections. The molecular basis for elevated IgM levels, neutropenia, or anemia has not been established.

Diagnosis

SSCP analysis of genomic DNA is diagnostic.

Counselling issues

IV immunoglobulin administration and prophylactic antibiotics can markedly reduce the number of infectious episodes. With current therapy, median age of death is 14 years.

Related conditions

A rare autosomal recessive form (MIM 605258) caused by mutation in the gene encoding the activation-induced cytidine deaminase (*AICDA*) gene on chromosome 12p13 has been described. *AICDA* plays an important role in the terminal differentiation of B cells.

References

Levy J, Espanol-Boren T, Thomas C, et al. Clinical spectrum of X-linked hyper-IgM syndrome. J Pediatr 1997;131:47–54.

Ramesh N, Geha RS, Notarangelo LD. CD40 ligand and the hyper-IgM syndrome. In: Ochs HD, Smith CIE, Puck JM, editors. Primary Immunodeficiency Diseases. New York: Oxford University Press; 1999. p. 233–49.

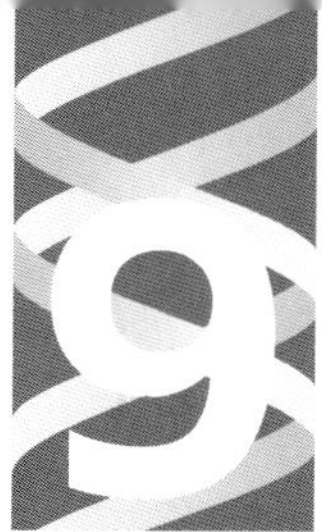

9. Neuromuscular diseases

Acid maltase deficiency **152**

Amyotrophic lateral sclerosis **154**

Congenital myasthenic syndromes **156**

Muscular dystrophy, Duchenne and Becker types **158**

Myotonic dystrophy **160**

Myotubular myopathy **162**

Nemaline myopathy **164**

Spinal muscular atrophy **166**

Acid Maltase Deficiency

(also known as: Glycogen storage disease type II; Alpha-1,4-glucosidase deficiency; Acid α-glucosidase deficiency; Pompe's disease [infantile-onset form])

MIM 232300

Clinical features

Infantile-onset disease

Patients often have respiratory muscle insufficiency that may lead to pulmonary infections. Other prominent manifestations include cardiomegaly, macroglossia, hepatomegaly, and generalized hypotonia and muscle weakness.

Adult-onset disease

The adult-onset form affects skeletal muscles more selectively. Progressive respiratory muscle weakness, predominantly of the diaphragm, is often the initial manifestation, with some patients presenting in respiratory failure. Pulmonary function tests show a reduced vital capacity, worse in the supine position, explaining the occasional complaint of orthopnea. Weakness in other muscles is more often proximal and in the lower extremities. Hepatomegaly and macroglossia have been reported rarely.

Age of onset The infantile-onset form presents by 1 year of age, and the adult-onset form after the second decade.

Epidemiology The prevalence is 1:138 000 for the infantile-onset form and 1:57 000 for the adult-onset form.

Inheritance Autosomal recessive

Chromosomal location 17q25.2–q25.3

Genes Acid maltase, or acid α-glucosidase, is a 105-kD protein encoded by the *GAA* gene, which encompasses 20 kb with over 20 exons. This lysosomal enzyme cleaves α-1,4- and α-1,6-glucosidic bonds in glycogen molecules.

Mutational spectrum

Missense, nonsense, and small deletion mutations are most common. A splice-site mutation in exon 1, a 536 bp deletion of exon 18 and part of a neighboring intron, and a single base-pair deletion at nucleotide 525 are the most frequent.

Effect of mutation

It is postulated that the infantile-onset form is due to mutations that cause almost complete absence of α-glucosidase protein or activity (e.g. deletion of exon 18). In contrast, it is thought that patients with the adult-onset form have one allele with some residual activity. Alleles associated with mild disease result in defective intracellular transport, inefficient post-translational processing, or altered tertiary structure.

Diagnosis

Creatinine kinase levels can be used for screening. It is recommended that α-glucosidase activity be measured in leukocytes and fibroblasts, followed by PCR analysis of restriction enzyme digestion to screen for the common mutations, or sequence analysis for more rare mutations.

Counselling issues

Death usually occurs by 1 year of age in the infantile form. Prenatal diagnosis can be made by amniocentesis.

Related conditions

There is a less common juvenile-onset form that manifests by the age of 15. Progressive respiratory muscle weakness usually leads to death by age 20 years.

References

Hirschhorn R. Glycogen storage disease type II: Acid α-glucosidase (acid maltase) deficiency. In: Scriver CR, Beaudet AL, Sly WS, Valle D, editors. The Metabolic and Molecular Basis of Inherited Disease. 8th ed. New York: McGraw-Hill; 2001. p. 3389–420.

Wokke JH, Ausems MG, van den Boogaard MJ, et al. Genotype-phenotype correlation in adult-onset acid maltase deficiency. Ann Neurol 1995;38 450–4.

Amyotrophic Lateral Sclerosis

(also known as: Lou Gehrig's disease; Charcot's disease; ALS)

MIM 105400

Clinical features Inspiratory and expiratory muscle weakness progresses from dyspnea to respiratory failure, the most common cause of death. Pulmonary function testing shows a decreased vital capacity, increased residual volume, normal total lung capacity, increased negative inspiratory pressure and decreased positive expiratory pressure. Bulbar involvement may cause vocal cord or other upper airway dysfunction, causing patients to become at risk of aspiration pneumonia. Upper and lower motor neuron dysfunction may first manifest as difficulty with manual dexterity or gait. Muscle weakness and cramps, fasciculations, hyperreflexia, pathologic reflexes, and bulbar signs develop later. Patients eventually develop hemiparesis or paraparesis. Sensory perception and autonomic function usually remain normal.

Age of onset Onset is in adulthood, and incidence increases with age.

Epidemiology The annual incidence rate for all types of ALS is 1–2.5:100 000. Five to ten percent of cases of ALS are familial.

Inheritance Autosomal dominant

Chromosomal location 22q12.2; 21q22.1; 18q21

Genes *SOD1*, with an mRNA of 560-bp, encodes the 32-kD Cu/Zn superoxide dismutase. Copper and zinc ions bind to the enzyme which then homodimerizes into its active form. The protein functions in the peroxisome to catalyze the conversion of harmful oxygen radicals into oxygen and hydrogen peroxide.

Mutational spectrum The vast majority of the more than 90 mutations are missense mutations that are distributed equally over the entire length of the gene. About half of all cases in North America are due to the missense mutation, A4V.

Effect of mutation The exact mechanisms by which mutations cause disease are unknown. The current hypothesis is that mutant superoxide dismutase uses peroxynitrite as a substrate to cause abnormal tyrosine nitration of various proteins, resulting in motor neuron cell death.

Diagnosis Diagnosis is made clinically by the presence of upper and lower motor neuron degeneration. Direct sequence analysis of cDNA can confirm the SOD1 mutation.

Counselling issues Death usually occurs 3–5 years after diagnosis, but individuals with onset earlier in life have a longer life expectancy. *SOD1* is responsible for only 20% of familial cases, and while other loci have been mapped, no other genes have been found.

Related conditions Two autosomal recessive forms of ALS exist: a juvenile form, ALS2 (MIM 205100), which maps to 2q33, and a non-juvenile form, ALS5 (MIM 602099), which maps to 15q15.1–q21.1. Other autosomal dominant forms include juvenile ALS4 on chromosome 9q34 (MIM 602433) and ALS with frontotemporal dementia (MIM 105550) on chromosome 9q21–q22.

References

Cole N, Siddique T. Genetic disorders of motor neurons. Semin Neurol 1999;19:407–18.

Rowland LP, Shneider NA. Amyotrophic lateral sclerosis. N Engl J Med 2001;344:1688–700.

Schiffman PL, Belsh JM. Pulmonary function at diagnosis of amyotrophic lateral sclerosis. Rate of deterioration. Chest 1993;103:508–13.

Congenital Myasthenic Syndromes

Type Ia

(also known as: Familial infantile myasthenia syndrome)

Type Ic

(also known as: Acetylcholinesterase deficiency syndrome)

Type Id

(also known as: Acetylcholine receptor deficiency syndrome)

Type IIa

(also known as: Slow channel syndrome)

MIM 601462

Clinical features Respiratory insufficiency, hypoxia, and apnea occur more frequently after continuous exertion. There are variable degrees of weakness, fatigability, and atrophy in all muscle groups that worsen with sustained contraction and fluctuate with time. Infants may have a poor suck reflex and difficulty feeding. All types show abnormal acetylcholine-dependent signaling at the neuromuscular junction.

Age of onset Onset usually occurs in infancy, but may not present until adulthood.

Epidemiology 1:500 000

Inheritance Autosomal recessive (Types Ia, Ic, and Id) and autosomal dominant with variable expressivity (Type IIa)

Chromosomal location COLQ; 17p13, 3p24.2
CHRNE; Chr. 17
CHRNA1; 2q24–q32
CHRNB1; 17p12–p11

Genes The gene in the 17p13 region, which causes Type Ia, has not been identified, but is postulated to encode synaptobrevin-2. *COLQ*, the gene for Type Ic on chromosome 3, encodes the collagen tail of the end-plate acetylcholinesterase that attaches acetylcholinestestase to the basal lamina. *CHRNE* on chromosome 17, the ϵ subunit of the acetylcholine receptor, can cause Types Id or IIa. *CHRNA1* on chromosome 2 and *CHRNB1* on chromosome 17, encoding the α and β subunits of the acetylcholine receptor, respectively, are also responsible for Type IIa.

Mutational spectrum

Most mutations in *COLQ* are nonsense, although frameshift insertions and deletions have also been reported. *CHRNE* mutations that cause Type Ic are due to premature terminations or missense mutations at essential residues. Type IIa is due to predominantly missense mutations in *CHRNE*, *CHRNA1*, and *CHRNB1*.

Effect of mutation

Synaptobrevin may cause Type Ia through defects in acetylcholine release from the presynaptic neuron. Mutations in *COLQ* prevent docking of acetylcholinesterase with the basal lamina. The acetylcholine receptor comprises two α, one β, one δ, and one ϵ subunit. Defects in the α, β, or ϵ subunits cause abnormal signal transmission from nerve to muscle.

Diagnosis

Direct sequencing of DNA is diagnostic.

Counselling issues

It is likely that defects in other genes can also cause disease.

References

Engel AG, Ohno K, Sine SM. Congenital myasthenic syndromes: recent advances. Arch Neurol 1999;56:163–7.

Engel AG. Myasthenic syndromes. In: Engel AG, Franzini-Armstrong C, editors. Myology. 2nd edition. New York: McGraw-Hill; 1994. p. 1798–835.

Muscular Dystrophy, Duchenne and Becker Type

(also known as: DMD; BMD)

MIM	310200
Clinical features	Progressive muscle weakness leads to respiratory dysfunction and ventilator dependence. Impaired mucus clearance can cause areas of atelectasis. Vital capacity decreases significantly with eventual development of hypercapnia. Nocturnal oxygen desaturation occurs in the more severe phenotypes. Scoliosis further reduces chest wall movement. Hip and lower limb muscle weakness, which cause gait difficulties, progress to atrophy of upper limbs and neck. Intellectual impairment is frequently present. BMD patients have a less severe phenotype.
Age of onset	Before age 3 years
Epidemiology	1:3000–4500 male births
Inheritance	X-linked recessive
Chromosomal location	Xp21.2, 12q21
Genes	The dystrophin gene, *DMD*, spans 79 exons over a 2.5-Mb region on the short arm of chromosome 21 and encodes a 427-kD protein. Dystrophin is part of the sarcolemma in skeletal muscle fibers.
Mutational spectrum	60% of dystrophin mutations are deletions, with most occurring in a proximal 800-kb or a central 200-kb region of the gene. About 1/3 of the mutations are thought to arise *de novo*.
Effect of mutation	The carboxy terminus of dystrophin interacts with β-dystroglycan, a membrane-bound protein that connects to laminin, the basal lamina, and other glycoproteins, while the amino terminus binds to actin. Dystrophin is absent in DMD and reduced or altered in BMD, leading to areas of muscle degeneration.

Diagnosis

Diagnosis is confirmed by PCR analysis of the hotspot deletion zones or quantitative Southern blotting after digestion with at least two restriction enzymes.

Counselling issues

Patients usually die in the third decade from respiratory infections. When patients inherit a spontaneous germline mutation from their mothers, the chance that another male sibling will develop the disease is approximately 15%. Prenatal screening can be accomplished by amniocentesis or chorionic villus biopsy.

Related conditions

X-linked dilated cardiomyopathy (MIM 302045), also due to mutations in the dystrophin gene, preferentially affects cardiac muscle.

References

Bakker E, van Ommen GJB. Duchenne and Becker muscular dystrophy (DMD and BMD). In: Emery AEH, editor. Neuromuscular Disorders: Clinical and Molecular Genetics. Chichester, England: John Wiley & Sons; 1998. p. 59–85.

Leger P, Leger SS. Respiratory concerns in Duchenne muscular dystrophy (DMD). Pediatr Pulmonol Suppl 1997;16:137–9.

Myotonic Dystrophy

(also known as: Dystrophia myotonica; Steinert's disease)

MIM	160900
Clinical features	Adult patients develop respiratory insufficiency due to weakness of the intercostal muscles, but central nervous system impairment can also limit respiratory drive. Muscle weakness, myotonia, cataracts, gonadal atrophy, and mild intellectual impairment are common. The congenital form has more severe neonatal respiratory distress, hypotonia, feeding difficulties, delayed motor development, and mental retardation.
Age of onset	The adult-onset form may present from adolescence through to the seventh decade. The congenital form presents soon after birth.
Epidemiology	1:8500
Inheritance	The adult-onset form is autosomal dominant with variable penetrance and anticipation, while congenital myotonic dystrophy is maternally transmitted.
Chromosomal location	19q13.2–q13.3
Genes	*DMPK*, the dystrophia myotonia protein kinase, spanning 15 exons over 13-kb of genomic DNA, encodes a 624-amino acid, 53-kD protein that is a putative serine-threonine protein kinase.
Mutational spectrum	The disease is caused by an increased number of CTG repeats in the 3′-untranslated exon. While unaffected individuals have up to 37 repeats, those with 37–49 repeats are considered to have premutations, and those with 50 to several thousand repeats have clinical disease.

Effect of mutation

The repeat expansion most likely causes a decreased amount of mRNA as a result of *DMPK* transcriptional downregulation. It is also postulated that the expansion alters chromatin structure and nucleosome binding, preventing translation of neighboring genes. Large expansions occur exclusively through the maternal line explaining why the congenital form is maternally transmitted.

Diagnosis

Southern blotting can demonstrate the number of CTG repeats. Greater than 50 repeats is consistent with clinical disease.

Counselling issues

In general, patients who inherit the mutation from their father are less severely affected. A positive correlation has been observed between the number of repeats and severity of disease.

References

Brewster B, Groenen P, Wieringa B. Myotonic dystrophy: clinical and molecular aspects. In: Emery AEH, editor. Neuromuscular Disorders: Clinical and Molecular Genetics. Chichester, England: John Wiley & Sons; 1998. p. 323–64.

Moxley RT. Myotonic muscular dystrophy. Handbook of Clinical Neurology 1992;18(62):209–59.

Myotubular Myopathy

(also known as: Centronuclear myopathy)

MIM 310400

Clinical features Profound muscle weakness at birth causes apnea requiring a ventilator. Patients often develop recurrent lung infections. Infants are often born prematurely with polyhydramnios noted *in utero*. Many affected individuals have ophthalmoplegia, swallowing difficulties, absent deep tendon reflexes, delayed motor development, characteristic facies, cryptorchidism, muscle contractures, and a lack of spontaneous muscle movements.

Age of onset Birth

Epidemiology Rare

Inheritance X-linked recessive

Chromosomal location Xq28

Genes *MTM1* spans 15 exons and encodes myotubularin, a member of the protein tyrosine phosphatase family. It dephosphorylates phosphatidylinositol 3-phosphate (PI(3)P), a second messenger involved in vesicular trafficking within muscle cells.

Mutational spectrum 133 mutations in approximately 200 families have been identified. Nonsense, missense, splice-site, and frameshift mutations are almost equally represented.

Effect of mutation The mutations in *MTM1* affect the ability of myotubularin to regulate the cellular levels of PI(3)P, which leads to disruption of myocyte differentiation, perhaps through altered vesicular trafficking.

Diagnosis Direct sequencing of the *MTM1* gene is diagnostic.

Counselling issues

More than 1/2 of patients die within the first year, but some have lived up to 10 years. Female carriers do not show any abnormalities.

Related conditions

There appear to be autosomal dominant and recessive forms of this disease that can be distinguished from the X-linked form by onset later in childhood and occurrence in females. The dominant form (MIM 160150) is due to a defect in the *MYF6* gene on chromosome 12 and is the least severe, whereas the recessive form (MIM 255200) is due to an unknown mutation and is intermediate in severity.

References

Herman GE, Finegold M, Zhao W, et al. Medical complications in long-term survivors with X-linked myotubular myopathy. J Pediatr 1999;134:206–14.

Laporte J, Biancalana V, Tanner SM, et al. MTM1 mutations in X-linked myotubular myopathy. Hum Mutat 2000;15:393–409.

Nemaline Myopathy

MIM 256030; 161800

Clinical features Respiratory muscle weakness may lead to respiratory insufficiency and ventilator dependence. Proximal muscle weakness is greater than distal and is most pronounced in the facial, neck flexor, and bulbar muscles, resulting in delayed development of motor skills. Vertebral abnormalities include hyperlordosis and scoliosis.

Age of onset Infancy

Epidemiology Rare

Inheritance Autosomal recessive (MIM 256030); autosomal dominant (MIM 161800)

Chromosomal location NEB; 2q22
ACTA1; 1q42.1
TPM3; 1q22–q23

Genes Located on chromosome 22, *NEB* encodes nebulin, a 6669-amino acid component of the matrix that is interspersed within the thick and thin filaments of muscle fibers. *ACTA1*, the gene that codes for the α chain of skeletal muscle actin, lies near the telomere on chromosome 1. Tropomyosin 3, encoded by *TPM3*, which is nearer to the centromere on chromosome 1, is a component of sarcomere thin filaments in slow, Type 1 muscle fibers.

Mutational spectrum Four frameshift, one nonsense, and one splice-site mutation have been found in *NEB*. Missense mutations in *ACTA1* can cause both autosomal recessive and dominant forms. A nonsense mutation at codon 31 in *TPM3* causes the autosomal recessive form, whereas the dominant form is due to a missense mutation at codon 9.

Effect of mutation

Mutations in all these proteins cause disruption of Z-disc formation in the sarcomeres of skeletal muscle.

Diagnosis

PCR-SSCP analysis of genomic DNA, followed by direct sequence analysis, is used to establish diagnosis.

Counselling issues

Most patients die within the first 2 years, but some survive later into childhood. There is possibly a fourth locus associated with this disease.

References

Wallgren-Pettersson C, Laing NG. Nemaline myopathy. In: Emery AEH, editor. Neuromuscular Disorders: Clinical and Molecular Genetics. Chichester, England: John Wiley & Sons; 1998. p. 247–62.

Wallgren-Pettersson C, Pelin K, Hilpela P, et al. Clinical and genetic heterogeneity in autosomal recessive nemaline myopathy. Neuromuscul Disord 1999;9:564–72.

Spinal Muscular Atrophy

(also known as: SMA I [Werdnig-Hoffman disease]; SMA II; SMA III [Kugelberg-Welander syndrome])

MIM

253300; 253550; 253400

Clinical features

Paralysis of the intercostal muscles causes abnormal respiration and ineffective clearance of airway secretions. Pulmonary hypoplasia results in decreased vital capacity. Absence of deep breaths leads to areas of atelectasis and increased functional residual capacity. Abnormal respirations cause rib cage deformity and scoliosis with progressive restriction. V/Q mismatches occur due to impaired ventilation. Patients develop hypoxia, and, depending on the degree of muscle paralysis, hypo-, normo-, or hyper-capnia. Pneumonia and respiratory insufficiency are often the cause of death. Other typical signs include proximal muscle weakness and atrophy, tongue fasciculations, and a positive Gower's sequence when attempting to stand.

Age of onset

Type I manifests in the first 6 months of life, Type II within the first year, and Type III by 3 years of age.

Epidemiology

SMA is the second most common lethal autosomal recessive genetic disorder. Type I occurs in 1:20 000, whereas Types II and III combined occur in 1:24 000.

Inheritance

Autosomal recessive

Chromosomal location

5q12.2–q13.3

Genes

SMN1, a survival motor neuron gene, has nine exons encoding a 294-amino acid protein that aids in the assembly of small nuclear ribonucleoprotein (snRNP) components. There is a second gene, *SMN2*, which is nearly identical and located adjacent to *SMN1* in an inverted duplication region. Only mutations in *SMN1*, however, result in disease.

Mutational spectrum

Approximately 95% of patients have a deletion of SMN1 exon 7 or exons 7 and 8. Over 20 other mutations have been identified.

Effect of mutation

SMN1 is found in high concentrations in spinal motor neurons. It is thought to interact with other neuron-specific proteins (e.g. neuron specific profilin II), and its absence results in degeneration of these cells. Deletions in a nearby gene, *NAIP*, are also found in a high percentage of patients, but its relationship to the phenotype is unknown.

Diagnosis

Diagnosis can be made by SSCP analysis of genomic DNA or PCR of exons 7 and 8 following restriction enzyme digestion.

Counselling issues

Death usually occurs within the first 2 years in Type I, during childhood in Type II, and in adulthood in Type III.

Related conditions

Diaphragmatic spinal atrophy, a variant of SMA I, is characterized by respiratory distress due to diaphragmatic paralysis. Inheritance is autosomal recessive with the gene localized to 11q13–q21.

References

Barois A, Estourret-Mathiaud B. Respiratory problems in spinal muscular atrophies. Pediatr Pulmonol Suppl 1997;16:140–1.

Wirth B. An update of the mutational spectrum of the survival motor neuron gene (SMN1) in autosomal recessive SMA. Hum Mutat 2000;15:228–37.

10. Other

Congenital central hypoventilation syndrome **170**

Klinefelter's syndrome **173**

Leigh disease **175**

Lung cancer **177**

Prader-Willi syndrome **179**

Rett syndrome **181**

Sarcoidosis **183**

Tuberous sclerosis **186**

Congenital Central Hypoventilation Syndrome

(also known as: Ondine's curse; Ondine-Hirschsprung disease; Congenital failure of autonomic control; CCHS)

MIM

209880

Clinical features

Patients exhibit normal ventilation while awake and alveolar hypoventilation while sleeping, although severe cases may also demonstrate daytime hypoventilation. Decreased tidal volume due to diminished chest wall motion with normal respiratory rate can lead to cyanosis. Patients have a decreased respiratory drive and decreased perception of asphyxia when challenged by hypercarbia or hypoxemia, but can maintain conscious control of breathing. Hirschsprung's disease, ganglioneuroma, neuroblastoma, ganglioneuroblastoma, diminished heart rate variability, and diminished pupillary light response are associated.

Age of onset

Infancy

Epidemiology

Rare, 160–180 cases known worldwide

Inheritance

Autosomal recessive, or autosomal dominant with reduced penetrance

Chromosomal location

EDN3; 20q13.2–q13.3
RET; 10q11.2
GDNF; 5p13.1–p12

Genes

The *EDN3* gene on chromosome 20 encodes the 238-amino acid precursor protein to endothelin 3. *RET*, a protooncogene from the receptor tyrosine kinase family, is located on chromosome 10 and contains 20 exons, encoding a 1114-amino acid protein. *GDNF*, the gene for glial cell line-derived neurotrophic factor on chromosome 5, encodes a 211-amino acid protein that is secreted as a 134-amino acid product that homodimerizes. It is likely that other genes can cause CCHS.

Mutational spectrum

Only one mutation has been reported in *EDN3*, a single nucleotide insertion in exon 5, leading to a frameshift and premature termination. Two missense mutations have been identified in *RET*, a threonine to alanine change in codon 706 and a proline to leucine substitution in codon 1039. An arginine to tryptophan missense mutation at codon 93 in *GDNF* has been found in one patient.

Effect of mutation

EDN3, *RET*, and *GDNF* are involved in neural crest cell and hindbrain development. Presumably, alterations in these genes cause abnormal growth, differentiation, or migration of these cells and subsequent abnormal ventilatory control.

Diagnosis

Respiratory physiology testing shows diminished response to endogenously or exogenously induced hypercarbia and hypoxemia while awake and asleep. Tidal volume, chest wall movement, oxygen saturation, and end-tidal carbon dioxide should also be measured.

Counselling issues

Patients need to have a tracheostomy for mechanical ventilation during sleep. Severely affected patients may need daytime mechanical ventilation or phrenic nerve stimulation for diaphragmatic pacing. Untreated, patients live for 1–2 months before the effects of chronic hypoxemia and hypercarbia are seen. Patients should be monitored in a center with expertise in CCHS.

Children should not be allowed to swim, but if they do, constant supervision is needed. Noncontact sports with moderate activity level and frequent resting should be encouraged.

Related conditions

Mutations in *EDN3* also cause isolated Hirschsprung's disease (MIM 142623) and Waardenburg-Shah syndrome (MIM 277580). *RET* mutations cause multiple endocrine neoplasia type IIA (MIM 171400) and type IIB (MIM 162300), medullary thyroid carcinoma (MIM 155240), and Hirschsprung's disease. *GDNF* mutations also cause Hirschsprung's disease.

References

Amiel J, Salomon R, Attie T, et al. Mutations of the RET-GDNF signaling pathway in Ondine's curse. Am J Hum Genet 1998;62:715–7.

Bolk S, Angrist M, Xie J, et al. Endothelin-3 frameshift mutation in congenital central hypoventilation syndrome. Nat Genet 1996;13:395–6.

Sakai T, Wakizaka A, Matsuda H, et al. Point mutation in exon 12 of the receptor tyrosine kinase proto-oncogene RET in Ondine-Hirschsprung syndrome. Pediatrics 1998;101:924–6.

American Thoracic Society. Idiopathic congenital central hypoventilation syndrome: diagnosis and management. Am J Respir Crit Care Med 1999;160:368–73.

Klinefelter's Syndrome

(also known as: KS)

MIM

145410

Clinical features

Patients tend to have a restrictive pattern with reduced functional residual capacity (FRC) and TLC on pulmonary function testing, presumably due to an abnormality of the chest wall. Other characteristics include gynecomastia, small testes, limited body hair, increased height and armspan:height ratio, androgen deficiency, and impaired spermatogenesis. There is also an increased risk of developing breast carcinoma, extragonadal germ cell tumors, autoimmune disorders, learning disabilities, psychiatric disorders, osteoporosis, and diabetes mellitus.

Age of onset

Disease is often first noticed at puberty.

Epidemiology

1:500 males

Chromosome findings

Patients most frequently have a 47,XXY karyotype, but 48,XXXY and 49,XXXXY are also possible. Due to mosaicism, not all cells have the abnormal chromosome number. For instance, buccal mucosal cells that can be used for karyotype analysis can be normal, while blood or testicular cells may have the extra chromosome.

Mechanism of inheritance

An extra X chromosome can be inherited in several different ways. One study found that disease occurred in 53.2% of patients because of paternal nondisjunction, 34.4% during maternal meiosis I, 9.3% during maternal meiosis II, and 3.2% due to post-mitotic errors in the zygote. Advanced maternal age increases the frequency of maternal meiosis I errors.

Effect of genetic anomaly

Patients have primary testicular failure with histologic changes such as hyalinization and fibrosis of the seminiferous tubules. Testosterone levels are low-normal in KS, but luteinizing hormone

(LH) production from the pituitary can be normal. Inhibin B, a product of Sertoli cells that is the presumed feedback regulator of follicule-stimulating hormone (FSH) at the pituitary, is markedly reduced.

Diagnosis

Demonstration of the XXY on karyotype is diagnostic.

Counselling issues

There is no increased risk of having another child with KS. Testosterone replacement instituted at age 11 or 12 years and continued for life can treat many of the features of androgen deficiency, but cannot correct infertility. Patients are unable to bear children due to absent spermatozoa. Gynecomastia can be corrected by plastic surgery.

References

Huseby JS, Petersen D. Pulmonary function in Klinefelter's syndrome. Chest 1981;80:31–3.

Smyth CM, Bremner WJ. Klinefelter syndrome. Arch Intern Med 1998;158:1309–14.

Leigh Disease

(also known as: Infantile subacute necrotizing encephalopathy)

MIM 256000

Clinical features Patients have ventilatory abnormalities due to central nervous system defects, manifested as apnea and/or irregular hyperpnea. Neurologic involvement includes encephalopathy, ataxia, intellectual regression, ophthalmoparesis, optic atrophy, hypotonia, and peripheral neuropathy. CT, magnetic resonance imaging (MRI), and autopsy findings show lesions throughout the basal ganglia, brainstem, and cerebellum. Failure to thrive is often the presenting sign. Hypertrophic cardiomyopathy and myopathy may be present.

Age of onset Symptoms present within months to years of birth.

Epidemiology Rare

Inheritance Autosomal recessive, X-linked, or maternal

Chromosomal location
SURF1; 9q34
NDUFV1 and *NDUFS8*; 11q13
NDUFS7; 19p13
PDHA1; Xp22.2-p22.1
MTATP6; mitochondrial DNA, nucleotides 8527–9207

Genes All genes encode components of the mitochondrial respiratory chain. *SURF1* on chromosome 9 produces a 1.0-kb cDNA that encodes the 300-amino acid surfeit-1 protein, a component of cytochrome c oxidase. *NDUFV1* on chromosome 11, with a 1.4-kb cDNA, encodes a 51-kD subunit of complex I, whereas *NDUFS8*, in the same region of chromosome 11, has seven exons spread over 6 kb of DNA that encodes the 23-kD subunit of complex I. *NDUFS7* on chromosome 19 encodes the 20-kD subunit of complex I. The E1α subunit of pyruvate dehydrogenase is the 361-amino acid product of the *PDHA1* gene on the X chromosome. Subunit 6 of ATP synthase is encoded by *MTATP6*, a 700-bp segment of mitochondrial DNA.

Mutational spectrum

About 20 mutations, mostly small deletions, have been found in *SURF1*. One missense and one nonsense mutation have been identified in *NDUFV1*, while two missense mutations are known in *NDUFS8*. The only mutation found in *NDUFS7* is missense ($V^{122}M$). A $D^{258}A$ mutation has been found in *PDAH1*. The sole mutations in *MTATP6* are nucleotide T8993 changing to cytosine or guanine.

Effect of mutation

All mutations result in defective production of ATP in mitochondria.

Diagnosis

Radiologic or pathologic identification of bilateral spongiform lesions in the basal ganglia, thalamus, and brain stem is used for diagnosis. Sequence analysis or PCR amplification with restriction enzyme digestion can provide confirmation.

Counselling issues

Death usually occurs in the first decade. Prognosis and prenatal diagnosis of the mitochondrial mutation is difficult because of heteroplasmy, the multiplicity of types of mitochondria in cells.

Related conditions

The Saguenay-Lac-Saint-Jean form (MIM 220111) of Leigh disease is named after a region in Quebec, Canada. The gene, localized to chromosome 2, is thought to be a subunit of cytochrome c oxidase. Other mutations in the mitochondrial genome ($A^{3243}G$ and $A^{8344}G$) may cause Leigh syndrome; mitochondrial myopathy, encephalopathy, lactic acidosis, and stroke-like episodes (MELAS) (MIM 540000); or myoclonic epilepsy associated with ragged red fibers (MERRF) (MIM 545000).

References

Dahl HH. Getting to the nucleus of mitochondrial disorders: identification of respiratory chain-enzyme genes causing Leigh syndrome. Am J Hum Genet 1998;63:1594–7.

Rahman S, Blok RB, Dahl HH, et al. Leigh syndrome: clinical features and biochemical and DNA abnormalities. Ann Neurol 1996;39:343–51.

Lung Cancer

MIM 211980

Age of onset Adulthood

Epidemiology Cancer of the lung is the second most common cancer, but has the highest mortality rate. Approximately 170 000 new cases are diagnosed per year with almost 160 000 deaths per year. The incidence is estimated at 73.7:100 000 in men and 43.0:100 000 in women. One in 12 males and one in 17 females will develop lung cancer. There is a higher incidence in African Americans than whites.

Inheritance Inheritance is polygenic and strongly influenced by environmental factors.

Genes Genes that predispose to lung cancer are often involved in the activation or detoxification of carcinogens, as shown in Table 3. Mutations in other genes, such as p53, k-Ras, and c-erbB2, are found in tumor cells, but not in somatic cells.

Counselling Issues Tobacco exposure is the most important risk factor for disease. Other risk factors include industrial exposures such as asbestos, radon, uranium, polycyclic aromatic hydrocarbons, and arsenic, and radiation exposure.

References

Bepler G. Lung cancer epidemiology and genetics. J Thorac Imaging 1999;14:228–34.

Haugen A, Ryberg D, Mollerup S, et al. Gene-environment interactions in human lung cancer. Toxicol Lett 2000;112-113:233–7.

Gene	Locus	Variants	Disease risk	Functional significance
Glutathione S-transferase M1 (GSTM1)	1p13.3	Homozygous deletion of entire gene	Greater odds of lung cancer	GSTM1 detoxifies carcinogenic compounds
Cytochrome P450IA1	15q22–q24	$I^{462}V$, presence of an Msp1 restriction site at nucleotide 264	Greater odds of lung cancer with either polymorphism. The risk is greater when one of these polymorphisms occurs with the GSTM1 deletion	P450 cytochromes detoxify polycyclic aromatic hydrocarbons in tobacco smoke, but products can be toxic. The $I^{462}V$ variant has greater enzymatic activity. The Msp1 polymorphism results in larger amounts of the enzyme
Cytochrome P450IIE1	10q24.3–qter	Absent RsaI restriction site in the 5'-flanking region	Greater odds of squamous cell cancer of the lung	This cytochrome, while detoxifying polycyclic aromatic compounds, also creates carcinogens
Myeloperoxidase	17q23.1	-463 G/A	Lower odds of lung cancer	Similar to the cytochromes, myeloperoxidase catalyzes reactions with carcinogenic end-products. Gene transcription is lower with this polymorphism
NAD(P)H: Quinone Oxidoreductase (NQO1)	16q22.1	$C^{609}T$	Greater odds of lung cancer	NQO1-catalyzed reactions also yield carcinogenic products

Table 3. Partial list of somatic gene polymorphisms that have been associated with disease risk.

Prader-Willi Syndrome

(also known as: Prader-Labhart-Willi syndrome; PWS)

MIM 176270

Clinical features Patients have abnormal responses to hypercapnia, hypoxia, and hyperoxia due to dysfunctional peripheral chemoreceptors. They also have obstructive sleep apnea due to the combination of obesity, muscle hypotonia, adenoidal and tonsillar hyperplasia, and narrow airways. Continuous positive airway pressure (CPAP) may be required during sleep to correct hypoxemia. Characteristic manifestations include dysmorphic facies, short stature, childhood obesity with hyperphagia, hypothalamic dysfunction, feeding difficulties in infancy, hypogonadism, muscle hypotonia, behavioral difficulties, and mental retardation.

Age of onset Neonatal period to infancy

Epidemiology 1:10 000–25 000

Inheritance The inheritance pattern is autosomal dominant, but most mutations arise *de novo*. Due to imprinting, mutations are only inherited from the father.

Chromosomal location 15q12; 15q11–q13; 15q11

Genes There are several candidate genes in the PWS critical region.

Mutational spectrum About 70% of cases are due to a large chromosomal deletion (about 4 Mb) in the paternal chromosome. Most other cases are caused by maternal uniparental disomy, in which both alleles in the region come from the mother. The result of both mechanisms is the absence of paternally-derived genes in the PWS critical region.

Normally, the promoter and first exon of one of the genes (*SNRPN*) in the critical region from the maternally-derived chromosome are hypermethylated, but the genes from the paternal chromosome are not. In addition, the shortest region of overlap of deletions from various patients with PWS includes the *SNRPN* gene. These findings indicate that *SNRPN* might be critical in the development of the disease.

Effect of mutation

Imprinting results from epigenetic modification of maternal and paternal chromosomes, usually through methylation. The mechanism by which *SNRPN* or any other gene in the PWS critical region causes disease is not understood.

Diagnosis

A scoring system based on clinical criteria has been used to establish diagnosis. Diagnosis can be confirmed by fluorescence *in situ* hybridization to detect the large deletion. PCR-based analysis of the parents and child can demonstrate uniparental disomy.

Counselling issues

Much of the management is directed toward behavioral modification. A low calorie diet, daily exercise, and limited access to food can reduce obesity. Group homes for adults with PWS are beneficial to manage behavioral and eating difficulties. The chance of having a second child with PWS is less than 1%.

Related conditions

Angelman syndrome (MIM 105830) is the counterpart of PWS, in which there is a large deletion in the maternally-derived chromosome or paternal uniparental disomy. It is characterized by abnormal facies, seizures, ataxia, mental retardation, and inappropriate laughter.

References

Cassidy SB. Prader-Willi syndrome. J Med Genet 1997;34:917–23.

Mann MR, Bartolomei MS. Towards a molecular understanding of Prader-Willi and Angelman syndromes. Hum Molec Genet 1999;8:1867–73.

Rett Syndrome

MIM 312750

Clinical features Patients exhibit a disordered ventilatory pattern when awake, characterized by intense hyperventilation punctuated by breath-holding spells with intermittent Valsalva-like maneuvers. Classically, patients have delayed growth of head circumference, impaired manual dexterity, psychomotor retardation, and gait dyspraxia. Other manifestations include air swallowing, a sporadic "creaking" bruxism, sleep disorders with night laughter, and screaming attacks.

Age of onset The first manifestations appear in early childhood, but the respiratory disorder usually begins in mid-childhood.

Epidemiology 1:15 000, almost all patients are female

Inheritance X-linked dominant

Chromosomal location Xq28

Genes The *MECP2* gene, which comprises four exons spanning 76 kb, encodes the methyl-CpG-binding protein-2 (MECP2) whose function is to repress transcription of methylated DNA regions by altering chromatin structure through deacetylation of histones. It has four putative domains: a methyl-CpG-binding domain, a transcriptional repression domain, and two nuclear localization-signal domains.

Mutational spectrum Most mutations are nonsense or frameshift, but four missense and four nonsense mutations represent about 65% of all mutations.

Effect of mutation Mutations in *MECP2* result in partial or complete loss of the inhibitory function of the protein. While the exact mechanism has not been elucidated, it is postulated that there is abnormal temporal regulation of gene expression during development, which may lead to aberrant neuronal connections.

Diagnosis

Diagnosis is confirmed by PCR-based sequence analysis of genomic DNA.

Counselling issues

Current PCR-based diagnostic methods may not be adequate to detect all mutations, particularly large deletions. Therefore, even if a mutation is not detected, the diagnosis of Rett syndrome is not excluded. Hemizygous males almost invariably die *in utero*. Prenatal testing can be completed by amniocentesis.

References

Dragich J, Houwink-Manville I, Schanen C. Rett syndrome: a surprising result of mutation in MECP2. Hum Mol Genet 2000;9:2365–75.

Hagberg B. Rett syndrome: clinical peculiarities and biological mysteries. Acta Paediatr 1995;84:971–6.

Kerr AM. A review of the respiratory disorder in the Rett syndrome. Brain Dev 1992;14:S43–5.

Sarcoidosis

MIM

181000

Clinical features

Presentation varies widely. Patients may complain of cough, dyspnea, and chest tightness. On physical examination, crackles may be auscultated and, rarely, clubbing may be evident. Other infrequent manifestations include pleural effusion, pneumothorax, and pleural thickening. Constitutional symptoms include weight loss, fatigue, and low-grade fever. Dermatologic manifestations consist of erythema nodosum and lupus pernio in acute and chronic disease, respectively. Uveitis is the most common ocular lesion, but other parts of the eye may be affected. Involvement of other organs may lead to peripheral lymphadenopathy, cardiac arrhythmias, abnormal liver function tests, anemia, leukopenia, arthritis, and hypercalcemia and hypercalciuria. The serum angiotensin-converting enzyme level is elevated in approximately half of patients. Chest X-ray may reveal hilar lymphadenopathy, pulmonary infiltrates, and, in advanced cases, fibrosis, bullae, and cysts.

Age of onset

Onset is usually in adulthood, most often before 40 years of age.

Epidemiology

1–40:100 000, but more prevalent in those of African descent. Females are affected slightly more often than males.

Inheritance

Development of sarcoidosis involves the interaction of genetic and environmental factors. Evidence to support this includes greater prevalence in certain racial and ethnic groups and familial aggregation.

Genes

Several studies have shown a familial inheritance pattern, but evidence for the identification of specific genes is conflicting. The human leukocyte antigen (HLA) genes have been studied most extensively, although not exclusively, as shown in Table 4. It is thought that the HLA genes may be involved through "molecular mimicry," as in ankylosing spondylitis, where antibodies against an antigen from an infectious organism are cross-reactive with a host HLA molecule. Alternative theories include the preferential binding of antigens from infectious organisms to certain HLA molecules or abnormal expression of HLA molecules leading to granulomata.

Other genes that may be related include *IL-1α*, which encodes a cytokine involved in the formation and maintenance of granulomata, and the genetic marker f13a*188 on 6p23–25, which is near the locus of interferon regulatory factor-4 (IRF4), a T cell attractant in granulomata.

Gene	Locus	Variants	Disease risk	Disease severity
HLA-A	6p21.3	*1	Greater	
HLA-B	6p21.3	*8	Greater	Less severe
HLA-DPB1	6p21.3	K69E	Greater	
HLA-DQB1	6p21.3	*0601		Greater incidence of cardiac sarcoidosis
HLA-DR	6p21.3	*3	Greater	Later onset, less severe course, greater incidence of arthritis
		*5, *6, *8	Greater	Earlier onset lacking eye involvement
		w52	Greater	More limited disease lacking eye involvement
		*17(3)		Less severe
		*14(6), *15(2), *16		More severe
Angiotensin converting enzyme	17q23	250-bp deletion in intron 16		Leads to higher ACE levels in certain patient populations, but does not cause disease
Chemokine (C-X3-C) receptor 1	3p21	V64I	Lower	
		32-bp deletion	Greater	
F13A genetic marker	6p25–p24	*188	Greater	
IL-1α genetic marker	2q13	*137	Greater	
TNF-β	6p21.3	*1		Worse course

Table 4. Partial list of genes that have been associated with disease risk or severity in sarcoidosis.

Diagnosis

Diagnosis is made by the presence of noncaseating granulomata on biopsy with appropriate clinical findings and the exclusion of other diseases with similar presentation. Transbronchial lung biopsy is often the preferred source of tissue for histological examination, but skin and lymph node biopsies may also be useful.

Counselling Issues

Spontaneous remission is most common, but 10–30% of patients have a chronic course. Mortality from sarcoidosis is 1–5%. The risk of developing sarcoidosis is greater for nonsmokers.

References

Statement on Sarcoidosis. Am J Respir Crit Care Med 1999;160:736–55.

Luisetti M, Beretta A, Casali L. Genetic aspects in sarcoidosis. Eur Respir J 2000;16:768–80.

Tuberous Sclerosis

(also known as: Tuberous sclerosis complex; TSC; Bourneville's disease)

MIM 191100

Clinical features Patients present with pulmonary lymphangioleiomyomatosis (LAM), abnormal smooth muscle proliferation that results in cyst formation, distortion of lung parenchyma, pneumothorax, dry cough, hemoptysis, and hypoxemia. Patients have multifocal micronodular pneumocyte hyperplasia (MMPH), a hamartomatous lesion of type II pneumocytes, and septal stroma with an increased number of macrophages. Seizures, adenoma sebaceum and other dermatologic manifestations, hamartomas in cardiac tissue, renal angiomyolipomas, mental retardation, and behavioral and psychological disorders are observed.

Age of onset Many manifestations appear in infancy to early childhood, but lung disease develops in adulthood.

Epidemiology The prevalence is 1–20:100 000. LAM occurs almost exclusively in women, affecting 30–40% of patients, but MMPH may occur in both men and women.

Inheritance Autosomal dominant

Chromosomal location *TSC1*; 9q34
TSC2; 16p13.3

Genes The *TSC1* gene on chromosome 9 has 23 exons and an 8.6-kb mRNA encoding the 130-kD hamartin protein, which is thought to function as a cell cycle regulator. Tuberin, a 1784-amino acid product of *TSC2* on chromosome 16, is a GTPase-activating protein (GAP) that acts as a tumor suppressor in cell growth and differentiation pathways. It has been suggested that hamartin and tuberin may interact in some common pathways.

Mutational spectrum

The most common mutations in *TSC1* are nonsense or deletions. *TSC2* mutations are mostly large deletions/rearrangements, small deletions, nonsense, or missense.

Effect of mutation

Most mutations in *TSC1* cause truncated proteins. *TSC2* mutations often result in truncated proteins or single amino acid replacements, frequently in exon 16 or 17 where the GAP domain is encoded. It is thought that these mutations cause disturbances in cell cycle regulation.

Diagnosis

The diagnosis of TSC is based on clinical criteria. Definite TSC requires the presence of two major criteria or one major and two minor criteria; probable TSC requires one major and one minor criteria; and possible TSC requires one major or two or more minor criteria. Major criteria are: facial angiofibromas or forehead plaque, nontraumatic ungual or periungual fibroma, three or more hypomelanotic macules, shagreen patch, multiple retinal nodular hamartomas, cortical tuber, subependymal nodule, subependymal giant cell astrocytoma, cardiac rhabdomyoma, and LAM or renal angiomyolipomas (AML). Minor criteria are: randomly distributed pits in dental enamel, hamartomatous rectal polyps, bone cysts, cerebral white matter radial migration lines, gingival fibromas, nonrenal hamartoma, retinal achromic patch, "confetti" skin lesions, and multiple renal cysts.

Counselling issues

Germline mosaicism has been described in several cases (i.e. when neither parent has a mutation, but their child is born with the disease). In these cases there is a 1–2% chance of having another child with TSC. About $^2/_3$ of TSC cases are due to sporadic mutations, most often in *TSC2*.

After diagnosis is made, a CT or MRI of the brain should be completed to look for cortical lesions, especially subependymal giant cell astrocytomas, and repeated every 1–3 years. Neurodevelopmental testing, ophthalmic examination, electrocardiogram (ECG), and renal ultrasound should also be completed. For adult females, chest CT should be completed to exclude LAM.

Related conditions

Sporadic LAM without evidence of TSC occurs in approximately 1:1 000 000, almost exclusively in young women, and is postulated to be due to mutations in both TSC2 alleles in somatic cells.

References

Carsillo T, Astrinidis A, Henske EP. Mutations in the tuberous sclerosis complex gene TSC2 are a cause of sporadic pulmonary lymphangioleiomyomatosis. Proc Natl Acad Sci USA 2000;97:6085–90.

Castro M, Shepherd CW, Gomez MR, et al. Pulmonary tuberous sclerosis. Chest 1995;107:189–95.

Cheadle JP, Reeve MP, Sampson JR, et al. Molecular genetic advances in tuberous sclerosis. Hum Genet 2000;107:97–114.

Hyman MH, Whittemore VH. National Institutes of Health consensus conference: tuberous sclerosis complex. Arch Neurol 2000;57:662–5.

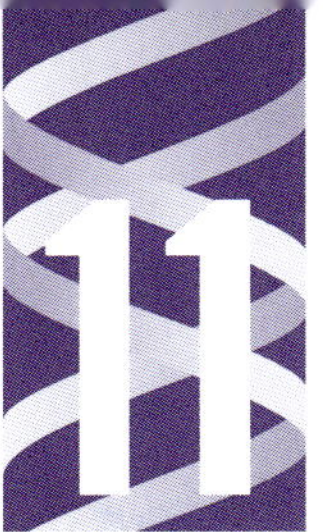

11. Abbreviations

A	Adenine
ADA	Adenosine deaminase
AIA	Aspirin-induced asthma
AICDA	Activation-induced cytidine deaminase
AML	Angiomyolipoma
AO II	Atelosteogenesis type II
APC	Activated protein C
APTT	Activated partial thromboplastin time
ASL	Airway surface liquid
AT	Ataxia telangiectasia
ATP	Adenosine triphosphate
AVM	Arteriovenous malformation
BCG	Bacillus Calmette-Guerin
bp	Basepair
C	Cytosine
cAMP	Cyclic adenosine monophosphate
CAP	Congenital alveolar proteinosis
cDNA	Complementary DNA
CF	Cystic fibrosis
CFTR	Cystic fibrosis transmembrane conductance regulator
chr.	Chromosome
COPD	Chronic obstructive pulmonary disease
CMV	Cytomegalovirus
CT	Computed tomography
dATP	Deoxyadenosine triphosphate
DC	Dyskeratosis congenita
D_LCO	Diffusion capacity of carbon monoxide
DNA	Deoxyribonucleic acid
ECG	Electrocardiogram
ELISA	Enzyme-linked immunosorbent assay
ENaC	Epithelial sodium channel
FEF_{25-75}	Forced expiratory flow 25–75%
FEV_1	Forced expiratory volume in 1 second
FHF	Familial Hibernian fever
FPF	Familial periodic fever
FRC	Functional residual capacity

FSH	Follicule-stimulating hormone
FVC	Forced vital capacity
G	Guanine
GAP	GTPase-activating protein
GM-CSF	Granulocyte-macrophage colony-stimulating factor
GTP	Guanosine triphosphate
HHT	Hereditary hemorrhagic telangiectasia
HLA	Human leukocyte antigen
HPS	Hermansky-Pudlak syndrome
Ig	Immunoglobulin
IL	Interleukin
IFN	Interferon
kb	Kilobase (10^3 nucleotides)
kD	Kilodalton
KS	Klinefelter syndrome
LAM	Lymphangioleiomyomatosis
LH	Luteinizing hormone
LTC_4	Leukotriene C_4
MAF	Macrophage-activating factor
Mb	Megabase (10^6 nucleotides)
MFS	Marfan syndrome
MHC	Major histocompatibility complex
MIM	Mendelian inheritance in man
MMPH	Multifocal micronodular pneumocyte hyperplasia
MRI	Magnetic resonance imaging
mRNA	Messenger RNA
NBD	Nucleotide-binding domain
NSAID	Nonsteroidal anti-inflammatory drug
PCR	Polymerase chain reaction
PGE2	Prostaglandin E_2
PHA	Phytohemagglutinins
PPD	Purified protein derivative
PWS	Prader-Willi syndrome
RAG	Recombination-activating gene
RDS	Respiratory distress syndrome
RNA	Ribonucleic acid

ROS	Reactive oxygen species
rRNA	Ribosomal RNA
RV	Residual volume
SCID	Severe combined immunodeficiency
SMA	Spinal muscle atrophy
snRNP	Small nuclear ribonucleoproteins
SSCP	Single-strand conformational polymorphism
T	Thymine
TAP	Transporter associated with antigen processing
TGF	Transforming growth factor
TLC	Total lung capacity
TNF	Tumor necrosis factor
TRAPS	TNF receptor-associated periodic syndromes
TSC	Tuberous sclerosis complex
VC	Vital capacity
V/Q	Ventilation/perfusion

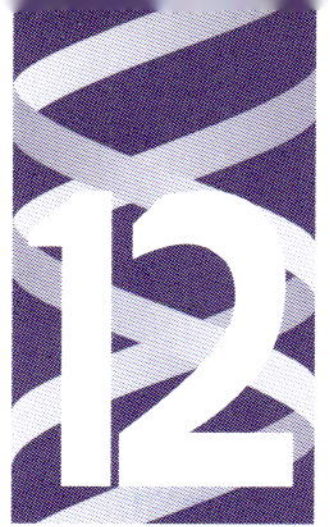

Glossary

A

Adenine (A)

One of the bases making up **DNA** and **RNA** (pairs with **thymine** in DNA and **uracil** in RNA).

Agarose gel electrophoresis

See **electrophoresis**

Allele

One of two or more alternative forms of a **gene** at a given location (**locus**). A single allele for each locus is inherited separately from each parent. In normal human beings there are two alleles for each locus (**diploidy**). If the two alleles are identical, the individual is said to be **homozygous** for that allele; if different, the individual is **heterozygous**.

For example, the normal **DNA** sequence at **codon** 6 in the beta-globin gene is GAG (coding for glutamic acid), whereas in sickle cell disease the sequence is GTG (coding for valine). An individual is said to be heterozygous for the glutamic acid → valine **mutation** if he/she possesses one normal (GAG) and one mutated (GTG) allele. Such individuals are **carriers** of the sickle cell gene and do not manifest classical sickle cell disease (which is **autosomal recessive**).

Allelic heterogeneity

Similar/identical **phenotypes** caused by different **mutations** within a **gene**. For example, many different mutations in the same gene are now known to be associated with Marfan's syndrome (*FBN1* gene at 15q21.1).

Amniocentesis

Withdrawal of amniotic fluid, usually carried out during the second trimester, for the purpose of prenatal diagnosis.

Amplification

The production of increased numbers of a **DNA** sequence.

1. *In vitro*
In the early days of recombinant DNA techniques, the only way to amplify a sequence of interest (so that large amounts were available

for detailed study) was to **clone** the fragment in a vector (**plasmid** or phage) and transform bacteria with the recombinant vector. The transformation technique generally results in the 'acceptance' of a single vector molecule by each bacterial cell. The vector is able to exist autonomously within the bacterial cell, sometimes at very high copy numbers (e.g. 500 vector copies per cell). Growth of the bacteria containing the vector, coupled with a method to recover the vector sequence from the bacterial culture, allows for almost unlimited production of a sequence of interest. Cloning and bacterial propagation are still used for applications requiring either large quantities of material or else exceptionally pure material.

However, the advent of the **polymerase chain reaction** (PCR) has meant that amplification of desired DNA sequences can now be performed more rapidly than was the case with cloning (a few hours cf. days), and it is now routine to amplify DNA sequences 10 million fold.

2. *In vivo*
Amplification may also refer to an increase in the number of DNA sequences within the genome. For example, the genomes of many tumors are now known to contain regions that have been amplified many fold compared to their non-tumor counterparts (i.e. a sequence or region of DNA that normally occurs once at a particular chromosomal location may be present in hundreds of copies in some tumors). It is believed that many such regions harbor **oncogenes**, which, when present in high copy number, predispose to development of the malignant **phenotype**.

Aneuploid

Possessing an incorrect number (abnormal complement) of **chromosomes**. The normal human complement is 46 chromosomes, any cell that deviates from this number is said to be aneuploid.

Aneuploidy

The chromosomal condition of a cell or organism with an incorrect number of **chromosomes**. Individuals with Down syndrome are described as having aneuploidy, because they possess an extra copy of chromosome 21 (**trisomy** 21), making a total of 47 chromosomes.

Anticipation

A general phenomenon that refers to the observation of an increase in severity, and/or decrease in age of onset, of a condition in successive generations of a family (see Figure 1). Anticipation is now known, in many cases, to result directly from the presence of a **dynamic mutation** in a family. In the absence of a dynamic mutation, anticipation may be explained by '**ascertainment bias**'. Thus, before the first dynamic mutations were described (in Fragile X and myotonic dystrophy), it was believed that ascertainment bias was the complete explanation for anticipation. There are two main reasons for ascertainment bias:

1. Identical **mutations** in different individuals often result in variable expressions of the associated **phenotype**. Thus, individuals within a family, all of whom harbor an identical mutation, may have variation in the severity of their condition.

2. Individuals with a severe phenotype are more likely to present to the medical profession. Moreover, such individuals are more likely to fail to reproduce (i.e. they are genetic lethals), often for social, rather than direct physical reasons.

For both reasons, it is much more likely that a mildly affected parent will be ascertained with a severely affected child, than the reverse. Therefore, the severity of a condition appears to increase through generations.

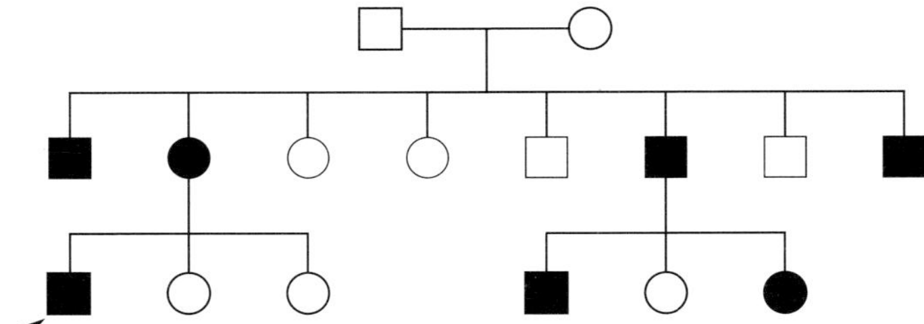

Figure 1. Autosomal dominant inheritance with **anticipation**. In many disorders that exhibit anticipation, the age of onset decreases in subsequent generations. It may happen that the transmitting parent (grandparent in this case) is unaffected at the time of presentation of the **proband** (see arrow). A good example is Huntington's disease, caused by the expansion of a CAG repeat in the coding region of the huntingtin gene. Note that this **pedigree** would also be consistent with either gonadal **mosaicism** or reduced **penetrance** (in the **carrier** grandparent).

Anticodon
The 3-base sequence on a **transfer RNA** (tRNA) molecule that is complementary to the 3-base **codon** of a **messenger RNA** (mRNA) molecule.

Ascertainment bias
See **anticipation**

Autosomal disorder
A disorder associated with a **mutation** in an autosomal **gene**.

Autosomal dominant (AD) inheritance
An **autosomal disorder** in which the **phenotype** is expressed in the **heterozygous** state. These disorders are not sex-specific. Fifty percent of offspring (when only one parent is affected) will usually manifest the disorder (Figure 2). Marfan syndrome is a good example of an AD disorder; affected individuals possess one wild-type (normal) and one mutated **allele** at the *FBN1* **gene**.

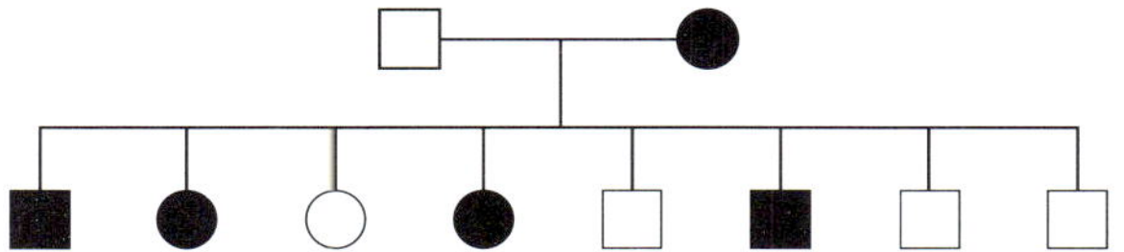

Figure 2. Autosomal dominant (AD) inheritance.

Autosomal recessive (AR) inheritance
An **autosomal disorder** in which the **phenotype** is manifest in the **homozygous** state. This pattern of inheritance is not sex-specific and is difficult to trace through generations because both parents must contribute the abnormal **gene**, but may not necessarily display the disorder. The children of two **heterozygous** AR parents have a 25% chance of manifesting the disorder (see Figure 3). Cystic fibrosis (CF) is a good example of an AR disorder; affected individuals possess two **mutations**, one at each **allele**.

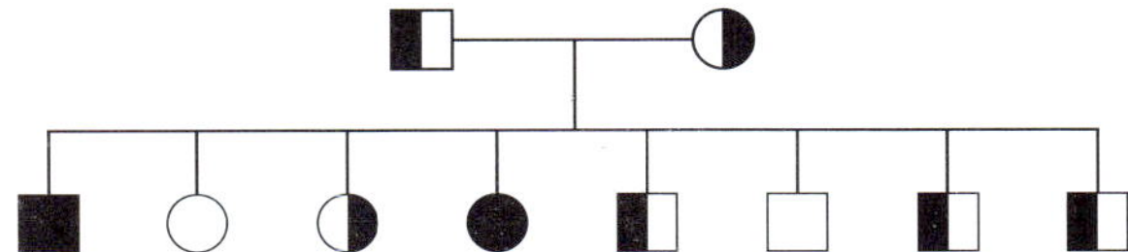

Figure 3. Autosomal recessive (AR) inheritance.

Autosome Any **chromosome**, other than the **sex chromosomes** (X or Y), that occurs in pairs in **diploid** cells.

B

Barr body An inactive **X chromosome**, visible in the **somatic cells** of individuals with more than one X chromosome (i.e. all normal females and all males with Klinefelter's syndrome). For individuals with n X chromosomes, n-1 Barr bodies are seen. The presence of a Barr body in cells obtained by **amniocentesis** or **chorionic villus sampling** used to be used as an indication of the sex of a baby before birth.

Base pair (bp) Two **nucleotides** held together by hydrogen bonds. In **DNA**, **guanine** always pairs with **cytosine**, and **thymine** with **adenine**. A base pair is also the basic unit for measuring DNA length.

C

Carrier An individual who is **heterozygous** for a mutant **allele** (i.e. carries one wild-type (normal copy) and one mutated copy of the **gene** under consideration).

CentiMorgan (cM) Unit of genetic distance. If the chance of **recombination** between two loci is 1%, the loci are said to be 1 cM apart. On average, 1 cM implies a physical distance of 1 Mb (1,000,000 **base pairs**) but significant deviations from this rule of thumb occur because recombination frequencies vary throughout the **genome**. Thus if recombination in a certain region is less likely than average, 1 cM may be equivalent to 5 Mb (5,000,000 base pairs) in that region.

Centromere Central constriction of the **chromosome** where daughter **chromatids** are joined together, separating the short (p) from the long (q) arms (Figure 4).

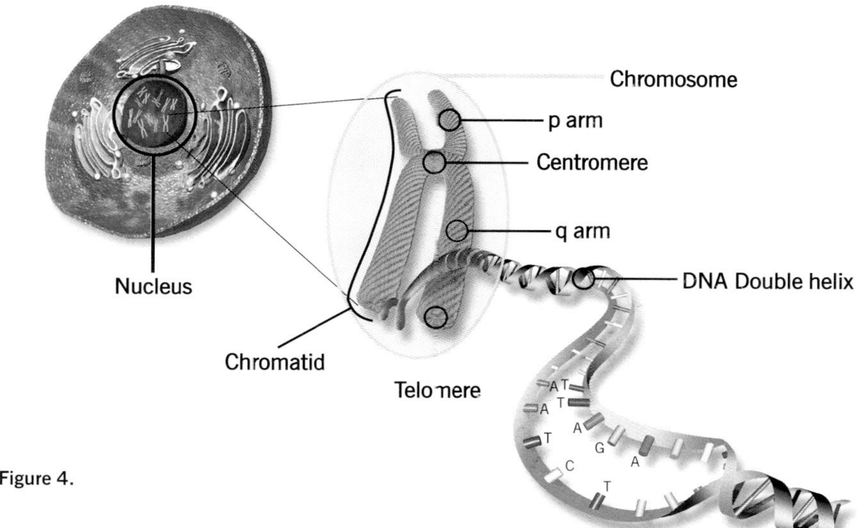

Figure 4.

Chorionic villus sampling (CVS)

Prenatal diagnostic procedure for obtaining fetal tissue at an earlier stage of gestation than **amniocentesis**. Generally performed after 10 weeks, ultrasound is used to guide aspiration of tissue from the villus area of the chorion.

Chromatid

One of the two parallel identical strands of a **chromosome**, connected at the **centromere** during **mitosis** and **meiosis** (see Figure 4). Before replication, each chromosome consists of only one chromatid. After replication, two identical sister chromatids are present. At the end of mitosis or meiosis, the two sisters separate and move to opposite poles before the cell splits.

Chromatin

A readily stained substance in the nucleus of a cell consisting of **DNA** and proteins. During cell division it coils and folds to form the metaphase **chromosomes**.

Chromosome

One of the threadlike 'packages' of **genes** and other **DNA** in the nucleus of a cell (see Figure 4). Humans have 23 pairs of chromosomes, 46 in total: 44 **autosomes** and two **sex chromosomes**. Each parent contributes one chromosome to each pair.

Chromosomal disorder A disorder that results from gross changes in **chromosome** dose. May result from addition or loss of entire chromosomes or just portions of chromosomes.

Clone A group of genetically identical cells with a common ancestor.

Codon A three-base coding unit of **DNA** that specifies the function of a corresponding unit (**anticodon**) of **transfer RNA** (tRNA).

Complementary DNA (cDNA) **DNA** synthesized from **messenger RNA** (mRNA) using **reverse transcriptase**. Differs from **genomic** DNA because it lacks **introns**.

Complementation The wild-type **allele** of a **gene** compensates for a mutant allele of the same gene so that the heterozygote's **phenotype** is wild-type.

Complementation analysis A genetic test (usually performed *in vitro*) that determines whether or not two **mutations** that produce the same **phenotype** are allelic. It enables the geneticist to determine how many distinct **genes** are involved when confronted with a number of mutations that have similar phenotypes.

Occasionally it can be observed clinically. Two parents who both suffer from **recessive** deafness (i.e. both are **homozygous** for a mutation resulting in deafness) may have offspring that have normal hearing. If A and B refer to the wild-type (normal) forms of the genes, and a and b the mutated forms, one parent could be aa, BB and the other AA, bb. If **allele**s A and B are distinct, each child will have the **genotype** aA, bB and will have normal hearing. If A and B are allelic, the child will be homozygous at this **locus** and will also suffer from deafness.

Compound heterozygote An individual with two different mutant **alleles** at the same **locus**.

Concordant A pair of twins who manifest the same **phenotype** as each other.

Consanguinity

Sharing a common ancestor, and thus genetically related. **Recessive** disorders are seen with increased frequency in consanguineous families.

Consultand

An individual seeking genetic advice.

Contiguous gene syndrome

A syndrome resulting from the simultaneous functional imbalance of a group of **genes** (see Figure 5). The nomenclature for this group of disorders is somewhat confused, largely as a result of the history of their elucidation. The terms submicroscopic rearrangement/deletion/duplication and micro-rearrangement/deletion/duplication are often used interchangeably. Micro or submicroscopic refer to the fact that such lesions are not detectable with standard cytogenetic approaches (where the limit of resolution is usually 10 Mb, and 5 Mb in only the most fortuitous of circumstances). A newer, and perhaps more comprehensive, term that is currently applied to this group of disorders is segmental aneusomy syndromes (SASs). This term embraces the possibility not only of loss or gain of a

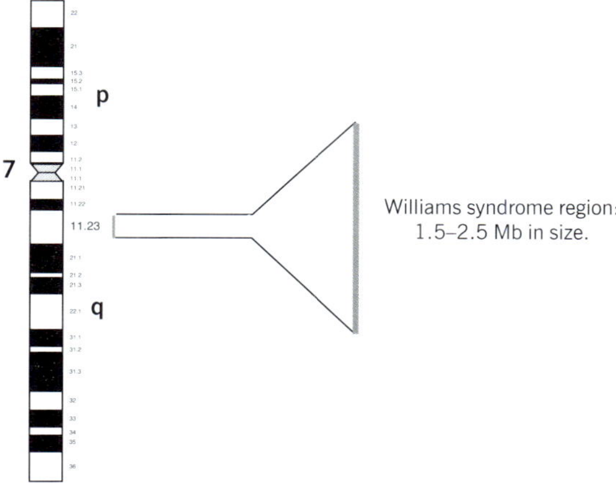

Figure 5. Schematic demonstrating the common deletion found in Williams syndrome, at 7q11.23. The common deletion is not detectable using standard cytogenetic analysis (even high resolution), despite the fact that the deletion is at least 1.5 Mb in size. In practice, only genomic rearrangements that affect at least 5–10 Mb are detectable, either by standard cytogenetic analysis or, in fact, any technique whose endpoint involves analysis at the chromosomal level. Such deletions are termed microdeletions or submicroscopic deletions. Approximately 20 genes are known to be involved in the 7q11.23 microdeletion, and work is underway to determine which genes contribute to which aspects of the Williams syndrome phenotype.

chromosomal region that harbors many genes (leading to imbalance of all those genes), but also of functional imbalance in a group of genes, as a result of an abnormality of the machinery involved in their silencing/**transcription** (i.e. methylation-based mechanisms that depend on a master control gene).

In practice, most contiguous gene syndromes result from the **heterozygous** deletion of a segment of **DNA** that is large in molecular terms but not detectable cytogenetically. The size of such deletions is usually 1.5–3 Mb. It is common for one to two dozen genes to be involved in such deletions, and the resultant **phenotypes** are often complex, involving multiple organ systems and, almost invariably, learning difficulties. A good example of a contiguous gene syndrome is Williams syndrome, a sporadic disorder that is due to a heterozygous deletion at **chromosome** 7q11.23. Affected individuals have characteristic phenotypes, including recognizable facial appearance and typical behavioral traits (including moderate learning difficulties). Velocardiofacial syndrome is currently the most common **microdeletion** known, and is caused by deletions of 3 Mb at chromosome 22q11.

Crossing over — Reciprocal exchange of genetic material between **homologous chromosomes** at **meiosis** (see Figure 6).

Cytogenetics — The study of the structure of **chromosomes**.

Cytosine (C) — One of the bases making up **DNA** and **RNA** (pairs with **guanine**).

Cytotrophoblast — Cells obtained from fetal chorionic villi by chorionic villus sampling (CVS). Used for **DNA** and **chromosome** analysis.

D

Deletion — A particular kind of **mutation** that involves the loss of a segment of **DNA** from a **chromosome** with subsequent re-joining of the two extant ends. It can refer to the removal of one or more bases within a **gene** or to a much larger aberration involving millions of bases. The

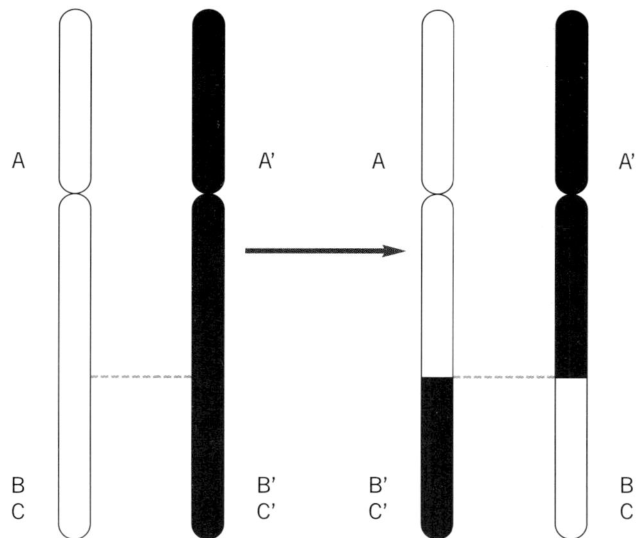

Figure 6. Schematic demonstrating the principle of **recombination (crossing over)**. On average, 50 recombinations occur per meiotic division (1–2 per **chromosome**). **Loci** that are far apart on the chromosome are more likely to be separated during recombination than those that are physically close to each other (they are said to be linked, see **linkage**), i.e. A and B are less likely to co-segregate than B and C. Note that the two **homologues** of a sequence have been differentially labeled according to their chromosome of origin.

term deletion is not totally specific, and differentiation must be made between **heterozygous** and **homozygous** deletions. Large heterozygous deletions are a common cause of complex **phenotypes** (see **contiguous gene syndrome**); large germ-line homozygous deletions are extremely rare but have been described. Homozygous deletions are frequently described in **somatic cells**, in association with the manifestation of the malignant phenotype. The two deletions in a homozygous deletion need not be identical but must result in the complete absence of DNA sequences that occupy the 'overlap' region.

Denature Broadly used to describe two general phenomena:

1. The 'melting' or separation of double-stranded **DNA** (dsDNA) into its constituent single strands, which may be achieved using heat or chemical approaches.

2. The denaturation of proteins. The specificity of proteins is a result of their 3-dimensional conformation, which is a function of their (linear) amino acid sequence. Heat and/or chemical approaches may result in denaturation of a protein—the protein loses its 3-dimensional conformation (usually irreversibly) and, with it, its specific activity.

Diploid

The number of **chromosomes** in most human **somatic cells** (46). This is double the number found in **gametes** (23, the **haploid** number).

Discordant

A pair of twins who differ in their manifestation of a **phenotype**.

Dizygotic

The fertilization of 2 separate eggs by 2 separate sperm resulting in a pair of genetically non-identical twins.

DNA (deoxyribonucleic acid)

The molecule of heredity. DNA normally exists as a double-stranded (ds) molecule; one strand is the complement (in sequence) of the other. The two strands are joined together by hydrogen bonding, a non-covalent mechanism that is easily reversible using heat or chemical means. DNA consists of 4 distinct bases: **guanine** (G), **cytosine** (C), **thymine** (T) and **adenine** (A). The convention is that DNA sequences are written in a 5' to 3' direction, where 5' and 3' refer to the numbering of carbons on the deoxyribose ring. A guanine on one strand will always pair with a cytosine on the other strand, while thymine pairs with adenine. Thus, given the sequence of bases on one strand, the sequence on the other is immediately determined:

5' – AGTGTGACTGATCTTGGTG – 3'
3' – TCACACTGACTAGAACCAC – 5'

The complexity (informational content) of a DNA molecule resides almost completely in the particular sequence of its bases. For a sequence of length 'n' **base pairs**, there are 4^n possible sequences. Even for relatively small n, this number is astronomical ($4n = 1.6 \times 10^{60}$ for n = 100).

The complementarity of the two strands of a dsDNA molecule is a very important feature and one that is exploited in almost all molecular genetic techniques. If dsDNA is **denatured**, either by heat or by chemical means, the two strands become separated from each other. If the conditions are subsequently altered (e.g. by reducing heat), the two strands eventually 'find' each other in solution and re-anneal to form dsDNA once again. The specificity of this reaction is quite high, under the right circumstances—strands that are not highly complementary are much less likely to re-anneal compared to perfect or near perfect matches. The process by which the two strands 'find' each other depends on random molecular collisions, and a '**zippering**' mechanism, which is initiated from a short stretch of complementarity. This property of DNA is vital for polymerase chain reaction (PCR), **Southern blotting** and any method that relies on the use of a DNA/**RNA probe** to detect its counterpart in a complex mix of molecules.

DNA chip

A 'chip' or microarray of multiple **DNA** sequences immobilized on a solid surface (see Figure 7). The term chip refers more often to semiconductor-based DNA arrays, in which short DNA sequences (oligos) are synthesized *in situ*, using a photolithographic process akin to that used in the manufacture of semiconductor devices for the electronics industry. The term microarray is much more general and includes any collection of DNA sequences immobilized onto a solid surface, whether by a photolithographic process, or by simple 'spotting' of DNA sequences onto glass slides.

The power of DNA microarrays is based on the parallel analysis that they allow for. In conventional **hybridization** analysis (i.e. **Southern blotting**), a single DNA sequence is usually used to interrogate a small number of different individuals. In DNA microarray analysis, this approach is reversed—an individual's DNA is hybridized to an array that may contain 30,000 distinct spots. This allows for direct information to be obtained about all DNA sequences on the array in one experiment. DNA microarrays have been used successfully to directly uncover **point mutations** in single **genes**, as well as detect

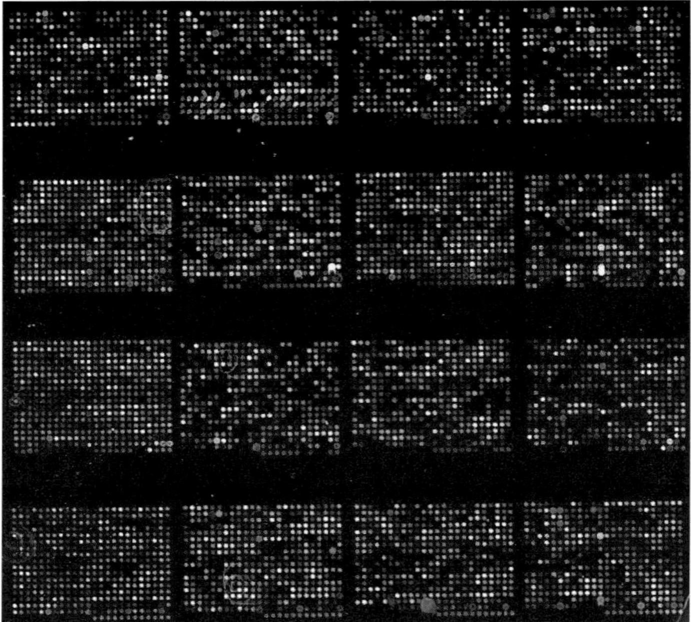

Figure 7. DNA chip. DNA arrays (or 'chips') are composed of thousands of 'spots' of DNA, attached to a solid surface (normally glass). Each spot contains a different DNA sequence. The arrays allow for massively parallel experiments to be performed on samples. In practice, two samples are applied to the array. One sample is a control (from a 'normal' sample) and one is the test sample. Each sample is labeled with fluorescent tags, control with green and test with red. The two labeled samples are co-hybridized to the array and the results read by a laser scanner. Spots on the array whose DNA content is equally represented in the test and control samples yield equal intensities in the red and green channels, resulting in a yellow signal. Spots appearing as red represent DNA sequences that are present at higher concentration in the test sample compared to the control sample and vice versa.

alterations in **gene expression** associated with certain disease states/cellular differentiation. It is likely that certain types of array will be useful in the determination of subtle copy number alterations, as occurs in **microdeletion/microduplication** syndromes.

DNA methylation

Addition of a methyl group (-CH_3) to **DNA nucleotides** (often **cytosine**). Methylation is often associated with reduced levels of expression of a given **gene** and is important in **imprinting**.

DNA replication

Use of existing **DNA** as a template for the synthesis of new DNA strands. In humans and other eukaryotes, replication takes place in the cell nucleus. DNA replication is semi-conservative—each new double-stranded molecule is composed of a newly synthesized strand and a pre-existing strand.

Dominant negative

A mutant **phenotype** in a heterozygote; the mutant **allele** exerts an effect despite there being only a single copy. Dominant negative effects cannot be corrected by the presence of a wild-type allele. The mechanism of dominance in this category varies but includes direct interference with the wild-type allele (for example, where both alleles participate in the formation of higher order structures). Another mechanism is a toxic effect on another cellular component, such as occurs in the polyglutamine disorders.

Dominant (traits/diseases)

Manifesting a **phenotype** in the **heterozygous** state. Individuals with Huntington's disease, a dominant condition, are affected even though they possess one normal copy of the **gene**.

Dynamic/ non-stable mutation

The vast majority of **mutations** known to be associated with human genetic disease are inter-generationally stable (no alteration in the mutation is observed when transmitted from parent to child). However, a recently described and growing class of disorders result from the presence of mutations that are unstable inter-generationally. These disorders result from the presence of tandem repeats of short **DNA** sequences (e.g. the sequence CAG may be repeated many times in tandem), see Table 1. For reasons that are not completely clear, the copy number of such repeats may vary from parent to child (usually resulting in a copy number increase) and within the **somatic cells** of a given individual. Abnormal **phenotypes** result when the number of repeats reaches a given threshold. Furthermore, when this threshold has been reached, the risk of even greater expansion of copy number in subsequent generations increases.

Disorder	Protein/location	Repeat	Repeat location	Normal range	Pre-mutation	Full mutation	Type	MIM
Progressive myoclonus epilepsy of Unverricht-Lundborg type (EPM1)	cystatin B 21q22.3	C_4GC_4G CG	Promoter	2-3	12-17	30-75	AR	254800
Fragile X type A (FRAXA)	FMR1 Xq27.3	CGG	5'UTR	6-52	~60-200	~200->2,000	XLR	309550
Fragile X type E (FRAXE)	FMR2 Xq28	CGG 5	C'UTR	6-25	-	>200	XLR	309548
Friedreich's ataxia (FRDA)	frataxin 9q13	GAA	intron	1 7-22	-	200- >900	AR	229300
Huntington's disease (HD)	huntingtin 4p16.3	CAG	ORF	6-34	-	36-180	AD	143100
Dentatorubal-pallidoluysian atrophy (DRPLA)	atrophin 12p12	CAG	ORF	7-25	-	49-88	AD	125370
Spinal and bulbar muscular atrophy (SBMA – Kennedy syndrome)	androgen receptor Xq11-12	CAG	ORF	11-24	-	40-62	XLR	313200
Spinocerebellar ataxia type 1 (SCA1)	ataxin-1 6p23	CAG	ORF	6-39	-	39-83	AD	164400
Spinocerebellar ataxia type 2 (SCA2)	ataxin-2 12q24	CAG	ORF	15-29	-	34-59	AD	183090
Spinocerebellar ataxia type 3 (SCA3)	ataxin-3 14q24.3-q31	CAG	ORF	13-36	-	55-84	AD	109150
Spinocerebellar ataxia type 6 (SCA6)	PQ calcium channel 19p13	CAG	ORF	4-16	-	21-30	AD	183086
Spinocerebellar ataxia type 7 (SCA7)	ataxin-7 3p21.1-p12	CAG	ORF	4-35	28-35	34- >300	AD	164500
Spinocerebellar ataxia type 8 (SCA8)	SCA8 13q21	CTG	3'UTR	6-37	-	~107-250[1]	AD	603680
Spinocerebellar ataxia type 10 (SCA10)	SCA10 22q13-qter	ATTCT	intron 9	10-22	-	500-4,500	AD	603516
Spinocerebellar ataxia type 12 (SCA12)	PP2R2B 5q31-33	CAG	5'UTR	7-28	-	66-78	AD	604326
Myotonic dystrophy (DM)	DMPK 19q13.3	CTG	3'UTR	5-37	~50-180	~200- >2,000	AD	160900

Table 1. 'Classical' repeat expansion disorders.

[1]Longer alleles exist but are not associated with disease.
AD: autosomal dominant; AR: autosomal recessive; ORF: open reading frame (coding region); 3' UTR: 3' untranslatec region (downstream of gene); 5' UTR: 5' untranslated region (upstream of gene); XLR: X-linked recessive.

E

Electrophoresis

The separation of molecules according to size and ionic charge by an electrical current.

Agarose gel electrophoresis
Separation, based on size, of **DNA/RNA** molecules through agarose. Conventional agarose gel electrophoresis generally refers to electrophoresis carried out under standard conditions, allowing the

resolution of molecules that vary in size from a few hundred to a few thousand **base pairs**.

Polyacrylamide gel electrophoresis
Allows resolution of proteins or DNA molecules differing in size by only 1 base pair.

Pulsed field gel electrophoresis
(Also performed using agarose) refers to a specialist technique that allows resolution of much larger DNA molecules, in some cases up to a few Mb in size.

Empirical recurrence risk – recurrence risk Based on observation, rather than detailed knowledge of, e.g., modes of inheritance or environmental factors.

Endonuclease An enzyme that cleaves **DNA** at an internal site (see also **restriction enzyme**).

Euchromatin **Chromatin** that stains lightly with trypsin G banding and contains active/potentially active **genes**.

Euploidy Having a normal **chromosome** complement.

Exon Coding part of a **gene**. Historically, it was believed that all of a **DNA** sequence is mirrored exactly on the messenger **RNA** (mRNA) molecule (except for the presence of **uracil** in mRNA compared to **thymine** in DNA). It was a surprise to discover that this is generally not the case. The **genomic** sequence of a gene has two components: exons and **introns**. The exons are found in both the genomic sequence and the mRNA, whereas the introns are found only in the genomic sequence. The mRNA for dystrophin, an **X-linked** gene associated with Duchenne muscular dystrophy (DMD), is 14,000 **base pairs** long but the genomic sequence is spread over a distance of 1.5 million base pairs, because of the presence of very long intronic sequences. After the genomic sequence is initially transcribed to RNA, a complex system ensures specific removal of introns. This system is known as **splicing**.

Expressivity Degree of expression of a disease. In some disorders, individuals carrying the same **mutation** may manifest wide variability in severity of the disorder. **Autosomal dominant** disorders are often associated with **variable expressivity**, a good example being Marfan's syndrome. Variable expressivity is to be differentiated from **incomplete penetrance**, an all or none phenomenon that refers to the complete absence of a **phenotype** in some **obligate carriers**.

F

Familial Any trait that has a higher frequency in relatives of an affected individual than the general population.

FISH Fluorescence *in situ* hybridization (see ***In situ* hybridization**).

Founder effect The high frequency of a mutant **allele** in a population as a result of its presence in a founder (ancestor). Founder effects are particularly noticeable in relative genetic isolates, such as the Finnish or Amish.

Frameshift mutation **Deletion/insertion** of a **DNA** sequence that is not an exact multiple of 3 **base pairs**. The result is an alteration of the reading frame of the **gene** such that all sequence that lies beyond the **mutation** is effectively nonsense (see Figure 8). A premature **stop codon** is usually encountered shortly after the frameshift.

G

Gamete (germ cell) The mature male or female reproductive cells, which contain a **haploid** set of **chromosomes**.

Gene An ordered, specific sequence of **nucleotides** that controls the transmission and expression of one or more traits by specifying the sequence and structure of a particular protein or **RNA** molecule. Mendel defined a gene as the basic physical and functional unit of all heredity.

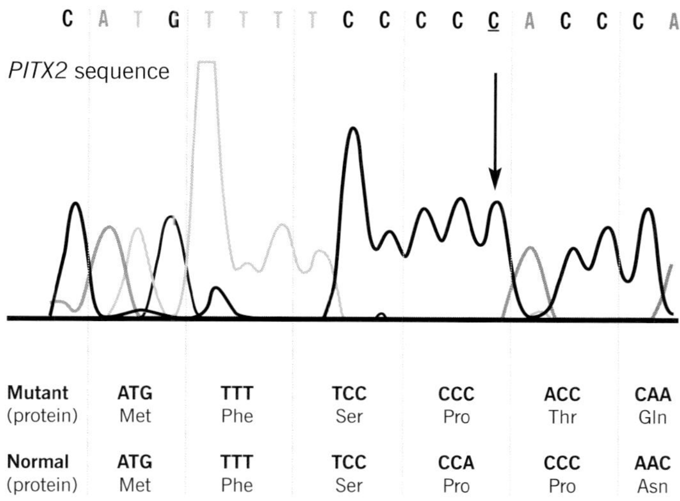

Figure 8. Frameshift mutation. This example shows a sequence of *PITX2* in a patient with Rieger's syndrome, an **autosomal dominant** condition. The sequence graph shows only the abnormal sequence. The arrow indicates the insertion of a single **cytosine** (C) residue. When translated the triplet code is now out of frame by one base pair. This totally alters the translated protein's amino acid sequence. This leads to a premature **stop codon** later in the protein and results in Rieger's syndrome.

Gene expression The process of converting a **gene's** coded information into the existing, operating structures in the cell.

Gene mapping Determines the relative positions of **genes** on a **DNA** molecule and plots the genetic distance in **linkage** units (**centiMorgans**) or physical distance (**base pairs**) between them.

Genetic code Relationship between the sequence of bases in a nucleic acid and the order of amino acids in the polypeptide synthesized from it (see Table 2). A sequence of three nucleic acid bases (a triplet) acts as a codeword (**codon**) for one amino acid or instruction (start/stop).

Genetic counselling Information/advice given to families with, or at risk of, genetic disease. Genetic counselling is a complex discipline that requires accurate diagnostic approaches, up-to-date knowledge of the genetics of the condition, an insight into the beliefs/anxieties/wishes

		2nd	2nd	2nd	2nd		
		T	C	A	G		
1st	T	TTT Phe [F]	TCT Ser [S]	TAT Tyr [Y]	TGT Cys [C]	T	3rd
		TTC Phe [F]	TCC Ser [S]	TAC Tyr [Y]	TGC Cys [C]	C	
		TTA Leu [L]	TCA Ser [S]	TAA Ter [end]	TGA Ter [end]	A	
		TTG Leu [L]	TCG Ser [S]	**TAG Ter [end]**	TGG Trp [W]	G	
1st	C	CTT Leu [L]	CCT Pro [P]	CAT His [H]	CGT Arg [R]	T	3rd
		CTC Leu [L]	CCC Pro [P]	CAC His [H]	CGC Arg [R]	C	
		CTA Leu [L]	CCA Pro [P]	CAA Gln [Q]	CGA Arg [R]	A	
		CTG Leu [L]	CCG Pro [P]	CAG Gln [Q]	CGG Arg [R]	G	
1st	A	ATT Ile [I]	ACT Thr [T]	AAT Asn [N]	AGT Ser [S]	T	3rd
		ATC Ile [I]	ACC Thr [T]	AAC Asn [N]	AGC Ser [S]	C	
		ATA Ile [I]	ACA Thr [T]	AAA Lys [K]	AGA Arg [R]	A	
		ATG Met [M]	ACG Thr [T]	AAG Lys [K]	AGG Arg [R]	G	
1st	G	GTT Val [V]	GCT Ala [A]	GAT Asp [D]	GGT Gly [G]	T	3rd
		GTC Val [V]	GCC Ala [A]	GAC Asp [D]	GGC Gly [G]	C	
		GTA Val [V]	GCA Ala [A]	GAA Glu [E]	GGA Gly [G]	A	
		GTG Val [V]	GCG Ala [A]	GAG Glu [E]	GGG Gly [G]	G	

Table 2. The **genetic code**. To locate a particular codon (e.g. TAG, marked in bold) locate the first base (T) in the left hand column, then the second base (A) by looking at the top row, and finally the third (G) in the right hand column (TAG is a stop codon). Note the redundancy of the genetic code—for example, three different codons specify a stop signal, and threonine (Thr) is specified by any of ACT, ACC, ACA and ACG.

of the individual seeking advice, intelligent risk estimation and, above all, skill in communicating relevant information to individuals from a wide variety of educational backgrounds. Genetic counselling is most often carried out by trained medical geneticists or, in some countries, specialist genetic counsellors or nurses.

Genetic heterogeneity

Association of a specific **phenotype** with **mutations** at different loci. The broader the phenotypic criteria, the greater the heterogeneity (e.g. mental retardation). However, even very specific phenotypes may be genetically heterogeneous. Tuberous sclerosis is a good example: this **autosomal dominant** condition is now known to be associated (in different individuals) with mutations either in the *TSC1* **gene** at 9q34 or the *TSC2* gene at 16p13.3. There is no obvious distinction between the clinical phenotypes associated with these two genes. **Genetic heterogeneity** should not be confused with **allelic heterogeneity**, which refers to the presence of different mutations at the same **locus**.

Genetic locus A specific location on a **chromosome**.

Genetic map A map of genetic landmarks deduced from **linkage** (**recombination**) **analysis**. Aims to determine the linear order of a set of **genetic markers** along a **chromosome**. Genetic maps differ significantly from **physical maps**, in that recombination frequencies are not identical across different **genomic** regions, resulting occasionally in large discrepancies.

Genetic marker A **gene** that has an easily identifiable **phenotype** so that one can distinguish between those cells or individuals that do or do not have the gene. Such a gene can also be used as a **probe** to mark cell nuclei or **chromosomes**, so that they can be isolated easily or identified from other nuclei or chromosomes later.

Genetic screening Population analysis designed to ascertain individuals at risk of either suffering or transmitting a genetic disease.

Genetically lethal Prevents reproduction of the individual, either because the condition causes death prior to reproductive age, or because social factors make it highly unlikely (although not impossible) that the individual concerned will reproduce.

Genome The complete **DNA** sequence of an individual, including the **sex chromosomes** and **mitochondrial DNA**. The genome of humans is estimated to have a complexity of 3.3×10^9 **base pairs** (per **haploid** genome).

Genomic Pertaining to the **genome**. Genomic **DNA** differs from **complementary DNA** in that it contains non-coding as well as coding DNA.

Genotype Genetic constitution of an individual, distinct from expressed features (**phenotype**).

Germ line Germ cells (those cells that produce **haploid gametes**) and the cells from which they arise. The germ line is formed very early in embryonic development. Germ line **mutations** are those present constitutionally in an individual (i.e. in all cells of the body) as opposed to somatic mutations, which affect only a proportion of cells.

Giemsa banding Light/dark bar code obtained by staining **chromosomes** with Giemsa stain. Results in a unique bar code for each chromosome.

Guanine (G) One of the bases making up **DNA** and **RNA** (pairs with **cytosine**).

H

Haploid The **chromosome** number of a normal **gamete**, containing one each of every individual chromosome (23 in humans).

Haploinsufficiency The presence of one active copy of a **gene**/region is insufficient to compensate for the absence of the other copy. Most genes are not 'haploinsufficient'—50% reduction of gene activity does not lead to an abnormal **phenotype**. However, for some genes, most often those involved in early development, reduction to 50% often correlates with an abnormal phenotype. Haploinsufficiency is an important component of most **contiguous gene disorders** (e.g. in Williams syndrome, **heterozygous deletion** of a number of genes results in the mutant phenotype, despite the presence of normal copies of all affected genes).

Hemizygous Having only one copy of a **gene** or **DNA** sequence in **diploid** cells. Males are hemizygous for most genes on the **sex chromosomes**, as they possess only one **X chromosome** and one **Y chromosome** (the exceptions being those genes with counterparts on both sex chromosomes). **Deletions** on **autosomes** produce hemizygosity in both males and females.

Heteroallelic The presence of distinct mutations at each **allele** of a given **locus/gene**.

Heterochromatin Contains few active **genes**, but is rich in highly repeated simple sequence **DNA**, sometimes known as satellite DNA. Heterochromatin refers to inactive regions of the **genome**, as opposed to **euchromatin**, which refers to active, gene expressing regions. Heterochromatin stains darkly with Giemsa.

Heteroplasmy The presence of two or more genetically distinct populations of mitochondrial genomes within a cell.

Heterozygote advantage Phenotypic advantage resulting from heterozygosity, this is not present in either wild-type or mutant homozygotes. An example is sickle cell anemia, those people that are **homozygous** for the wild-type **allele** (AA) have normal O_2 transport but are susceptible to malaria, those who are homozygous for the mutant allele (SS) have severely reduced O_2 transport but are resistant to malaria. Heterozygotes (AS) display the advantages from both alleles; they have nearly normal O_2 transport and are resistant to malaria.

Heterozygous Presence of two different **alleles** at a given **locus**.

Histones Simple proteins bound to **DNA** in **chromosomes**. They help to maintain **chromatin** structure and play an important role in regulating **gene** expression.

Holandric Pattern of inheritance displayed by **mutations** in **genes** located only on the **Y chromosome**. Such mutations are transmitted only from father to son.

Homologue or homologous gene Two or more **genes** whose sequences manifest significant similarity because of a close evolutionary relationship. May be between species (orthologues) or within a species (paralogues).

Homologous chromosomes **Chromosomes** that pair during **meiosis**. These chromosomes contain the same linear **gene** sequences as one another and derive from one parent.

Homology Similarity in **DNA** or protein sequences between individuals of the same species or among different species.

Homozygous Presence of identical **alleles** at a given **locus**.

Human gene therapy The study of approaches to treatment of human genetic disease, using the methods of modern molecular genetics. Many trials are underway studying a variety of disorders including cystic fibrosis. Some disorders are likely to be more treatable than others—it is probably going to be easier to replace defective or absent **gene** sequences rather than deal with genes whose aberrant expression results in an actively toxic effect.

Human genome project Worldwide collaboration aimed at obtaining a complete sequence of the human **genome**. Most sequencing has been carried out in the USA, although the Sanger Centre in Cambridge, UK has sequenced one third of the genome, and centers in Japan and Europe have also contributed significantly. The first draft of the human genome was released in the summer of 2000 to much acclaim. The finished sequence may not be available until 2003. Celera, a privately funded venture, headed by Dr Craig Ventner, also published its first draft at the same time.

Hybridization Pairing of complementary strands of nucleic acid. Also known as **re-annealing**. May refer to re-annealing of **DNA** in solution, on a membrane (**Southern blotting**) or on a DNA microarray. May also be used to refer to fusion of two **somatic cells**, resulting in a hybrid that contains genetic information from both donors.

I

Imprinting A general term used to describe the phenomenon whereby a **DNA** sequence (coding or otherwise) carries a signal or imprint that indicates its parent of origin. For most DNA sequences, no distinction can be made between those arising paternally and those arising maternally (apart from subtle sequence variations); for imprinted sequences this is not the case. The mechanistic basis of imprinting is almost always methylation—for certain **genes**, the copy that has been inherited from the father is methylated, while the maternal copy is not. The situation may be reversed for other imprinted genes. Note that imprinting of a gene refers to the general phenomenon, not which parental copy is methylated (and, therefore, usually inactive). Thus, formally speaking, it is incorrect to say that a gene undergoes paternal imprinting. It is correct to say that the gene undergoes imprinting and that the inactive (methylated) copy is always the paternal one. However, in common genetics parlance, paternal imprinting is usually understood to mean the same thing.

***In situ* hybridization** Annealing of **DNA** sequences to immobilized **chromosomes**/cells/tissues. Historically done using radioactively labeled **probes**, this is currently most often performed with fluorescently tagged molecules (fluorescent *in situ* hybridization – **FISH**, see Figure 9). ISH/FISH allows for the rapid detection of a DNA sequence within the **genome**.

Incomplete penetrance Complete absence of expression of the abnormal **phenotype** in a proportion of individuals known to be **obligate carriers**. To be distinguished from **variable expressivity**, in which the phenotype always manifests in obligate carriers but with widely varying degrees of severity.

Index case – proband The individual through which a family medically comes to light. For example, the index case may be a baby with Down syndrome. Can be termed propositus (if male) or proposita (if female).

Insertion Interruption of a chromosomal sequence as a result of insertion of material from elsewhere in the **genome** (either a different **chromosome**, or elsewhere from the same chromosome). Such insertions may result in abnormal **phenotypes** either because of direct interruption of a **gene** (uncommon), or because of the resulting imbalance (i.e. increased dosage) when the chromosomes that contain the normal counterparts of the inserted sequence are also present.

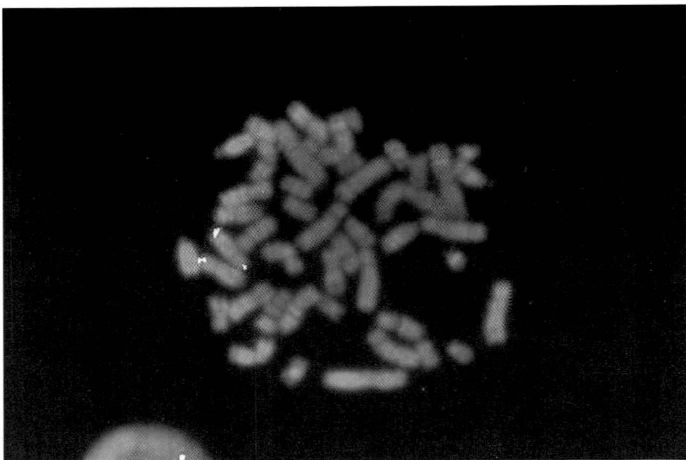

Figure 9. Fluorescence *in situ* hybridization. FISH analysis of a patient with a complex syndrome, using a clone containing **DNA** from the region 8q24.3. In addition to that clone, a control from 8pter was used. The 8pter clone has yielded a signal on both **homologues** of **chromosome** 8, while the 'test' clone from 8q24.3 has yielded a signal on only one homologue, demonstrating a (**heterozygous**) deletion in that region.

Intron

A non-coding **DNA** sequence that 'interrupts' the protein-coding sequences of a **gene**; intron sequences are transcribed into **messenger RNA** (mRNA) but are cut out before the mRNA is translated into a protein (this process is known as **splicing**). Introns may contain sequences involved in regulating expression of a gene. Unlike the **exon**, the intron is the **nucleotide** sequence in a gene that is not represented in the amino acid sequence of the final gene product.

Inversion

A structural abnormality of a **chromosome** in which a segment is reversed, as compared to the normal orientation of the segment. An inversion may result in the reversal of a segment that lies entirely on one chromosome arm (paracentric) or one that spans (i.e. contains) the **centromere** (pericentric). While individuals who possess an inversion are likely to be genetically balanced (and therefore usually phenotypically normal), they are at increased risk of producing unbalanced offspring because of problems at **meiosis** with pairing of the inversion chromosome with its normal **homologue**. Both

deletions and duplications may result, with concomitant congenital abnormalities related to **genomic** imbalance, or miscarriage if the imbalance is lethal.

K

Karyotype A photomicrograph of an individual's **chromosomes** arranged in a standard format showing the number, size, and shape of each chromosome type, and any abnormalities of chromosome number or morphology (see Figure 10).

Kilobase (kb) 1000 **base pairs** of **DNA**.

Knudson hypothesis See **tumor suppressor gene**

L

Linkage Co-inheritance of **DNA** sequences/**phenotypes** as a result of physical proximity on a **chromosome**. Before the advent of molecular genetics, linkage was often studied with regard to proteins, enzymes or cellular characteristics. An early study demonstrated linkage between the Duffy blood group and a form of **autosomal dominant** congenital cataract (both are now known to reside at 1q21.1). Phenotypes may also be linked in this manner (i.e. families manifesting two distinct Mendelian disorders).

During the **recombination** phase of **meiosis**, genetic material is exchanged (equally) between two **homologous chromosomes**. **Genes**/DNA sequences that are located physically close to each other are unlikely to be separated during recombination. Sequences that lie far apart on the same chromosome are more likely to be separated. For sequences that reside on different chromosomes, segregation will always be random, so that there will be a 50% chance of two markers being co-inherited.

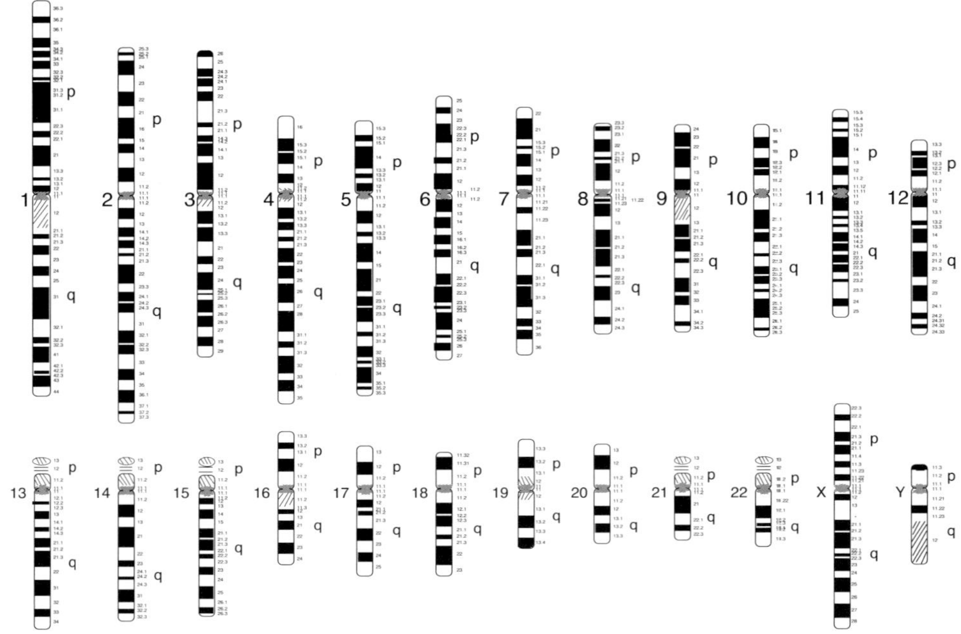

Figure 10. Schematic of a normal human (male) **karyotype**. (ISCN 550 ideogram produced by the MRC Human Genetics Unit, Edinburgh, reproduced with permission.)

Linkage analysis

An algorithm designed to map (i.e. physically locate) an unknown **gene** (associated with the **phenotype** of interest) to a chromosomal region. Linkage analysis has been the mainstay of disease-associated gene identification for some years. The general availability of large numbers of DNA markers that are variable in the population (**polymorphisms**), and which therefore permit **allele** discrimination, has made linkage analysis a relatively rapid and dependable approach (see Figure 11). However, the method relies on the ascertainment of large families manifesting Mendelian disorders. Relatively little phenotypic heterogeneity is tolerated, as a single misassigned individual (believed to be unaffected despite being a gene **carrier**) in a **pedigree** may completely invalidate the results. **Genetic heterogeneity** is another problem, not within

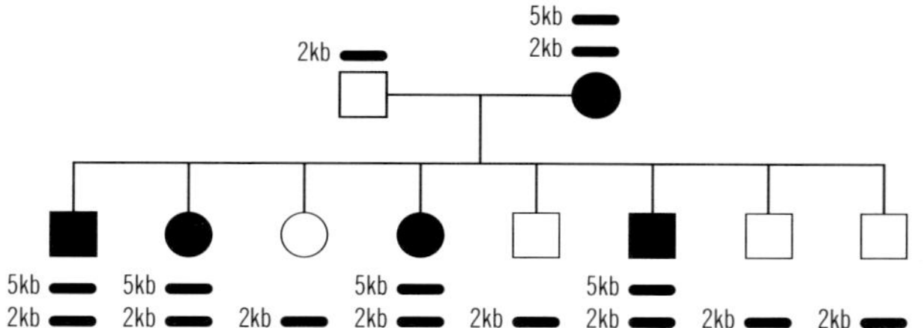

In the example above, note that the (affected) mother has a 5 kb band in addition to a 2 kb band. All the unaffected individuals have the small band only, all those who are affected have the large band. The unaffected individuals must have the mother's 2 kb fragment rather than her 5 kb fragment, and the affected individuals must have inherited the 5 kb band from the mother (as the father does not have one)—note that those individuals who only show the 2 kb band still have two alleles (one from each parent), they are just the same size and so cannot be differentiated. Thus, it appears that the 5 kb band is segregating with the disorder. The results in a family such as this are suggestive but further similar results in other families would be required for a sufficiently high **LOD** score.

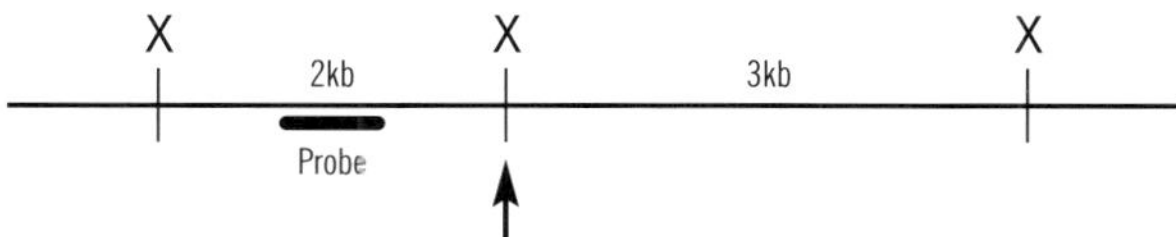

The **probe** recognizes a **DNA** sequence adjacent to a restriction site (see arrow) that is polymorphic (present on some **chromosomes** but not others). When such a site is present, the **DNA** is cleaved at that point and the probe detects a 2 kb fragment. When absent, the DNA is not cleaved and the probe detects a fragment of size (2 + 3) kb = 5 kb. X refers to the points at which the **restriction enzyme** will cleave the DNA. The recognition sequence for most restriction enzymes is very stringent—change in just one **nucleotide** will result in failure of cleavage. Most RFLPs result from the presence of a single nucleotide polymorphism that has altered the restriction site.

Figure 11. Schematic demonstrating the use of **restriction fragment length polymorphisms** (RFLPs) in **linkage analysis.**

families (usually) but between families. Thus, conditions that result in identical phenotypes despite being associated with **mutations** within different genes (e.g. tuberous sclerosis) are often hard to study. Linkage analysis typically follows a standard algorithm:

1. Large families with a given disorder are ascertained. Detailed clinical evaluation results in assignment of affected vs. unaffected individuals.

2. Large numbers of polymorphic DNA markers that span the **genome** are analyzed in all individuals (affected and unaffected).

3. The results are analyzed statistically, in the hope that one of the markers used will have demonstrably been co-inherited with the phenotype in question more often than would be predicted by chance.

The LOD score (**logarithm of the odds**) gives an indication of the likelihood of the result being significant (and not having occurred simply as a result of chance co-inheritance of the given marker with the condition).

Linkage disequilibrium Association of particular **DNA** sequences with each other, more often than is likely by chance alone (see Figure 12). Of particular relevance to inbred populations (e.g. Finland), where specific disease **mutations** are found to reside in close proximity to specific variants of DNA markers, as a result of the **founder effect**.

Linkage map A map of **genetic markers** as determined by genetic analysis (i.e. **recombination** analysis). May differ markedly from a map determined by actual physical relationships of genetic markers, because of the variability of recombination.

Locus The position of a **gene/DNA** sequence on the **genetic map**. Allelic genes/sequences are situated at identical loci in **homologous chromosomes**.

Locus heterogeneity **Mutations** at different loci cause similar **phenotypes**.

LOD (Logarithm of the Odds) score A statistical test of **linkage**. Used to determine whether a result is likely to have occurred by chance or to truly reflect linkage. The LOD score is the logarithm (base 10) of the likelihood that the linkage is meaningful. A LOD score of 3 implies that there is only a 1:1000 chance that the results have occurred by chance (i.e. the result would be likely to occur once by chance in 1000 simultaneous

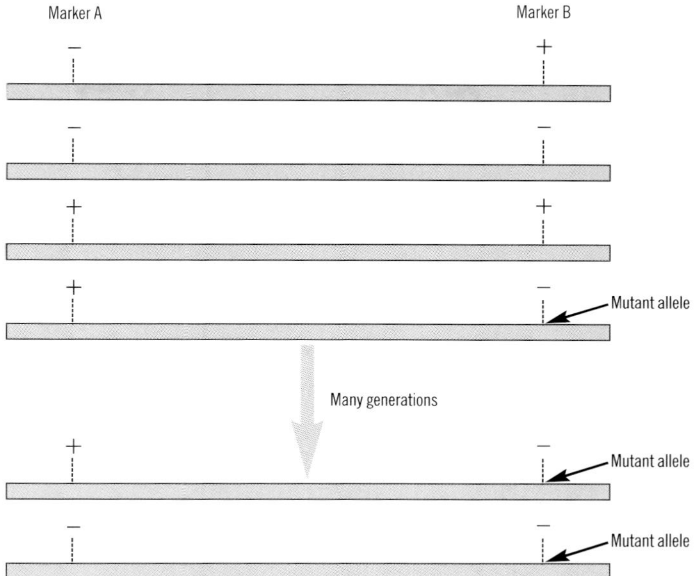

A **gene** is physically very close to marker B and further from marker A. Markers A and B, both on the same **chromosome**, can exist in one of two forms : +/-. Thus there are 4 possible **haplotypes**, as shown. If the **founder** mutation in the gene occurred as shown, then it is likely that even after many generations the mutant **allele** will segregate with the – form of marker B, as **recombination** is unlikely to have occurred between the two. However, since marker A is further away, the gene will now often segregate with the – form of marker A, which was not present on the original chromosome. The likelihood of recombination between the gene and marker A will depend on the physical distance between them, and on rates of recombination. It is possible that the gene would show a lesser but still significant degree of linkage disequilibrium with marker A.

Figure 12. Schematic demonstrating the concept of **linkage disequilibrium**.

studies addressing the same question). This is taken as proof of linkage (see Figure 11).

Lyonisation The inactivation of n-1 **X chromosomes** on a random basis in an individual with n X chromosomes. Named after Mary Lyon, this mechanism ensures dosage compensation of **genes** encoded by the X chromosome. X chromosome inactivation does not occur in normal males who possess only one X chromosome but does occur in one of the two X chromosomes of normal females. In males who possess more than one X chromosome (i.e. XXY, XXXY, etc.), the rule is the same and only one X chromosome remains active. X-inactivation occurs in early embryonic development and is random in each cell. The inactivation pattern in each cell is faithfully maintained in all daughter cells. Therefore, females are genetic **mosaics**, in that they possess two populations of cells with respect to the X chromosome: one population has one X active, while in the other population the other X is active. This is relevant to the expression of **X-linked** disease in females.

M

Maternal triple screen Measurement of unconjugated estrogen, α-fetoprotein, and human chorionic gonadotrophin during pregnancy for the purpose of reducing the risk of Down syndrome in mothers deemed too young (<35 years) for invasive prenatal tests (such as amniocentesis).

Meiosis The process of cell division by which male and female **gametes** (germ cells) are produced. Meiosis has two main roles. The first is **recombination** (during meiosis I). The second is reduction division. Human beings have 46 **chromosomes**, and each is conceived as a result of the union of two germ cells; therefore, it is reasonable to suppose that each germ cell will contain only 23 chromosomes (i.e. the **haploid** number). If not, then the first generation would have 92 chromosomes, the second 184, etc. Thus, at meiosis I, the number of chromosomes is reduced from 46 to 23.

Mendelian inheritance Refers to a particular pattern of inheritance, obeying simple rules: each **somatic cell** contains 2 **genes** for every characteristic and each pair of genes divides independently of all other pairs at **meiosis**.

Mendelian Inheritance in Man (MIM/OMIM) A catalogue of human Mendelian disorders, initiated in book form by Dr Victor McKusick of Johns Hopkins Hospital in Baltimore, USA. The original catalogue (produced in the mid-1960s) listed approximately 1500 conditions. By December 1998, this number had risen to 10,000, at the time of writing (November 2001) the figure had reached 13,118. With the advent of the Internet, MIM is now available as an online resource, free of charge (OMIM – Online Mendelian Inheritance in Man). The URL for this site is: http://www.ncbi.nlm.nih.gov/omim/. The online version is updated regularly, far faster than is possible for the print version, therefore, new **gene** discoveries are quickly assimilated into the database. OMIM lists disorders according to their mode of inheritance:

1 ---- (100000-) **Autosomal dominant** (entries created before May 15, 1994)

2 ---- (200000-) **Autosomal recessive** (entries created before May 15, 1994)

3 ---- (300000-) **X-linked** loci or **phenotypes**

4 ---- (400000-) Y-linked loci or phenotypes

5 ---- (500000-) Mitochondrial loci or phenotypes

6 ---- (600000-) Autosomal loci/phenotypes (entries created after May 15, 1994).

Full explanations of the best way to search the catalogue are available at the home page for OMIM.

Messenger RNA (mRNA) The template for protein synthesis, carries genetic information from the nucleus to the ribosomes where the code is translated into protein. Genetic information flows: **DNA** → RNA → protein.

Methylation See **DNA methylation**

Microdeletion Structural **chromosome** abnormality involving the loss of a segment that is not detectable using conventional (even high resolution) cytogenetic analysis. Microdeletions usually involve 1–3 Mb of sequence (the resolution of cytogenetic analysis rarely is better than 10 Mb). Most microdeletions are **heterozygous**, although some individuals/families have been described with **homozygous** microdeletions. See also **contiguous gene syndrome**.

Microduplication

Structural **chromosome** abnormality involving the gain of a segment that may involve long sequences (commonly 1–3 Mb), which are, nevertheless, undetectable using conventional cytogenetic analysis. Patients with microduplications have 3 copies of all sequences within the duplicated segment, as compared to 2 copies in normal individuals. See also **contiguous gene syndrome**.

Microsatellites

DNA sequences composed of short tandem repeats (STRs), such as di- and trinucleotide repeats, distributed widely throughout the **genome** with varying numbers of copies of the repeating units. Microsatellites are very valuable as **genetic markers** for mapping human **genes**.

Missense mutation

Single base substitution resulting in a **codon** that specifies a different amino acid than the wild-type.

Mitochondrial disease/disorder

Ambiguous term referring to disorders resulting from abnormalities of mitochondrial function. Two separate possibilities should be considered.

1. **Mutations** in the mitochondrial **genome** (see Figure 13). Such disorders will manifest an inheritance pattern that mirrors the manner in which mitochondria are inherited. Therefore, a mother will transmit a mitochondrial mutation to all her offspring (all of whom will be affected, albeit to a variable degree). A father will not transmit the disorder to any of his offspring.

2. Mutations in nuclear encoded **genes** that adversely affect mitochondrial function. The mitochondrial genome does not code for all the genes required for its maintenance, many are encoded in the nuclear genome. However, the inheritance patterns will differ markedly from the category described in the first option, and will be indistinguishable from standard Mendelian disorders.

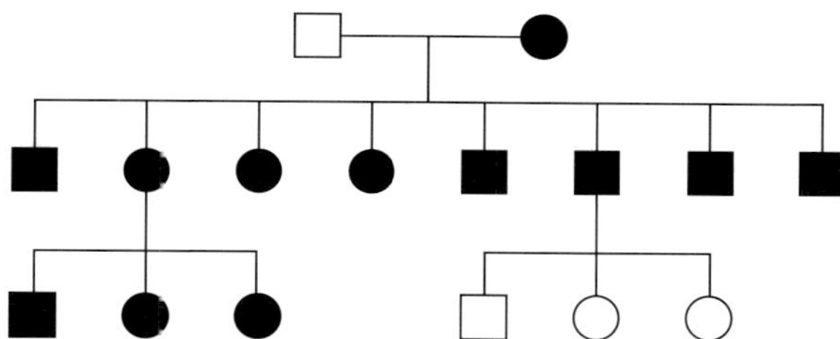

Figure 13. Mitochondrial inheritance. This **pedigree** relates to mutations in the mitochondrial **genome**.

Each mitochondrion possesses between 2–10 copies of its genome, and there are approximately 100 mitochondria in each cell. Therefore, each cell possesses 200–1000 copies of the mitochondrial genome. Heteroplasmy refers to the variability in sequence of this large number of genomes—even individuals with mitochondrial genome mutations are likely to have wild-type **alleles**. Variability in the proportion of molecules that are wild-type may have some bearing on the clinical variability often seen in such disorders.

Mitochondrial DNA The **DNA** in the circular **chromosome** of mitochondria. Mitochondrial DNA is present in multiple copies per cell and mutates more rapidly than **genomic** (nuclear) DNA.

Mitosis Cell division occurring in **somatic cells**, resulting in two daughter cells that are genetically identical to the parent cell.

Monogenic trait Causally associated with a single **gene** (see Mendelian trait).

Monosomy Absence of one of a pair of **chromosomes**.

Monozygotic Arising from a single **zygote** or fertilized egg. Monozygotic twins are genetically identical.

Mosaicism or mosaic Refers to the presence of two or more distinct cell lines, all derived from the same **zygote**. Such cell lines differ from each other as a result of **DNA** content/sequence. Mosaicism arises when the genetic alteration occurs post-fertilization (post-zygotic). The important features that need to be considered in mosaicism are:

The proportion of cells that are 'abnormal'. In general, the greater the proportion of cells that are abnormal, the greater the severity of the associated **phenotype**.

The specific tissues that contain high levels of the abnormal cell line(s). This variable will clearly also be relevant to the manifestation of any phenotype. An individual may have a **mutation** bearing cell line in a tissue where the mutation is largely irrelevant to the normal functioning of that tissue, with a concomitant reduction in phenotypic sequelae.

Mosaicism may be functional, as in normal females who are mosaic for activity of the two **X chromosomes** (see **Lyonisation**).

Mosaicism may occasionally be observed directly. **X-linked** skin disorders, such as incontinentia pigmenti, often manifest **mosaic** changes in the skin of a female, such that abnormal skin is observed alternately with normal skin, often in streaks (Blaschko's lines), which delineate developmental histories of cells.

Multifactorial inheritance — A type of hereditary pattern resulting from a complex interplay of genetic and environmental factors.

Mutation — Any heritable change in **DNA** sequence.

N

Non-disjunction — Failure of two **homologous chromosomes** to pull apart during **meiosis** I, or two **chromatids** of a chromosome to separate in meiosis II or **mitosis**. The result is that both are transmitted to one daughter cell, while the other daughter cell receives neither.

Non-dynamic (stable) mutations Stably inherited **mutations**, in contradistinction to **dynamic mutations**, which display variability from generation to generation. Includes all types of stable mutation (single base substitution, small **deletions/insertions**, **microduplications** and **microdeletions**).

Non-penetrance Failure of expression of a **phenotype** in the presence of the relevant **genotype**.

Nonsense mutation A single base substitution resulting in the creation of a **stop codon** (see Figure 14).

Northern blot **Hybridization** of a radio-labeled **RNA/DNA probe** to an immobilized RNA sequence. So called in order to differentiate it from **Southern blotting** which was described first. Neither has any relationship to points on the compass. Southern blotting was named after its inventor Ed Southern (currently Professor of Biochemistry at Oxford University, UK).

Nucleotide A basic unit of **DNA** or **RNA** consisting of a nitrogenous base—**adenine**, **guanine**, **thymine** or **cytosine** in DNA, and adenine, guanine, **uracil** or cytosine in RNA. A nucleotide is composed of a phosphate molecule, and a sugar molecule—deoxyribose in DNA and ribose in RNA. Many thousands or millions of nucleotides link to form a DNA or RNA molecule.

O

Obligate carrier See **obligate heterozygote**

Obligate heterozygote (obligate carrier) An individual who, on the basis of **pedigree** analysis, must carry the mutant **allele**.

Oncogene A **gene** that, when over expressed, causes neoplasia. In contrast to **tumor suppressor genes**, which result in tumorigenesis when their activity is reduced.

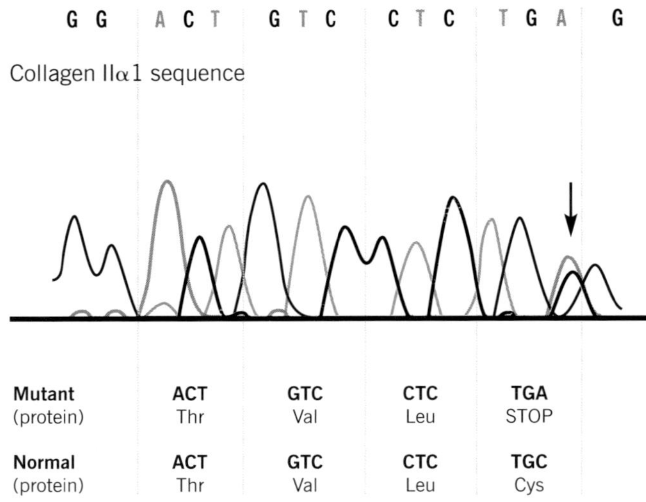

Figure 14. Nonsense mutation. This example shows a sequence graph of collagen II (alpha 1) in a patient with Stickler syndrome, an **autosomal dominant** condition. The sequence is of **genomic DNA** and shows both normal and abnormal sequences (the patient is heterozygous for the mutation).
The base marked with an arrow has been changed from C to A. When translated the codon is changed from TGC (cysteine) to TGA (stop). The premature **stop codon** in the collagen gene results in Stickler syndrome.

P

p Short arm of a **chromosome** (from the French *petit*) (see Figure 4).

Palindromic sequence A **DNA** sequence that contains the same 5' to 3' sequence on both strands. Most **restriction enzymes** recognize palindromic sequences. An example is 5' – AGATCT – 3', which would read 3' – TCTAGA – 5' on the complementary strand. This is the recognition site of *Bgl*II.

Pedigree A schematic for a family indicating relationships to the **proband** and how a particular disease or trait has been inherited (see Figure 15).

Penetrance An all-or-none phenomenon related to the proportion of individuals with the relevant **genotype** for a disease who actually manifest

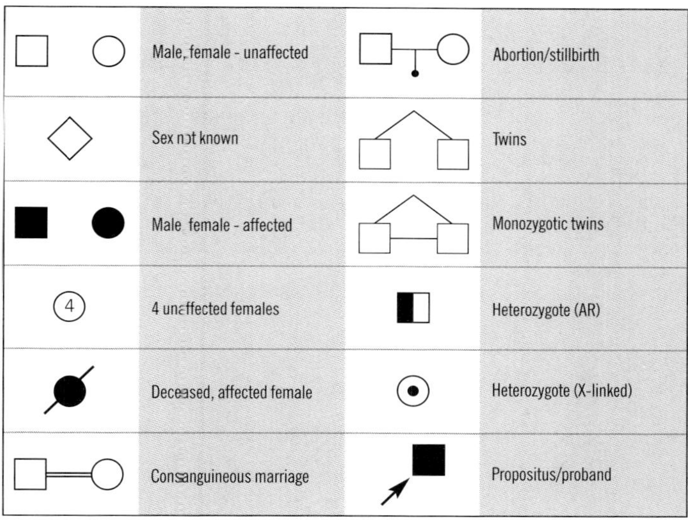

Figure 15. Symbols commonly used in **pedigree** drawing.

the **phenotype**. Note the difference between penetrance and **variable expressivity**.

Phenotype Observed disease/abnormality/trait. An all-embracing term that does not necessarily imply pathology. A particular phenotype may be the result of **genotype**, the environment or both.

Physical map A map of the locations of identifiable landmarks on **DNA**, such as specific DNA sequences or **genes**, where distance is measured in **base pairs**. For any **genome**, the highest resolution map is the complete **nucleotide** sequence of the **chromosomes**. A physical map should be distinguished from a **genetic map**, which depends on **recombination** frequencies.

Plasmid Found largely in bacterial and protozoan cells, plasmids are autonomously replicating, extrachromosomal, circular **DNA** molecules that are distinct from the normal bacterial **genome** and are often used as vectors in recombinant DNA technologies. They are not essential for cell survival under non-selective conditions, but can be incorporated into the genome and are transferred between cells if they encode a protein that would enhance survival under selective conditions (e.g. an enzyme that breaks down a specific antibiotic).

Pleiotropy Diverse effects of a single **gene** on many organ systems (e.g. the **mutation** in Marfan's syndrome results in lens dislocation, aortic root dilatation and other pathologies).

Ploidy The number of sets of **chromosomes** in a cell. Human cells may be **haploid** (23 chromosomes, as in mature sperm or ova), **diploid** (46 chromosomes, seen in normal **somatic cells**) or triploid (69 chromosomes, seen in abnormal somatic cells, which results in severe congenital abnormalities).

Point mutation Single base substitution.

Polygenic disease Disease (or trait) that results from the simultaneous interaction of multiple **gene** mutations, each of which contributes to the eventual **phenotype**. Generally, each **mutation** in isolation is likely to have a relatively minor effect on the phenotype. Such disorders are not inherited in a Mendelian fashion. Examples include hypertension, obesity and diabetes.

Polymerase chain reaction (PCR) A molecular technique for amplifying **DNA** sequences *in vitro* (see Figure 16). The DNA to be copied is **denatured** to its single strand form and two synthetic oligonucleotide primers are annealed to complementary regions of the target DNA in the presence of excess deoxynucleotides and a heat-stable DNA polymerase. The power of PCR lies in the exponential nature of **amplification**, which results from repeated cycling of the 'copying' process. Thus, a single molecule will be copied in the first cycle, resulting in 2 molecules. In the second cycle, each of these will also be copied, resulting in 4 copies. In theory, after n cycles, there will be 2^n molecules for each starting molecule. In practice, this theoretical limit is rarely

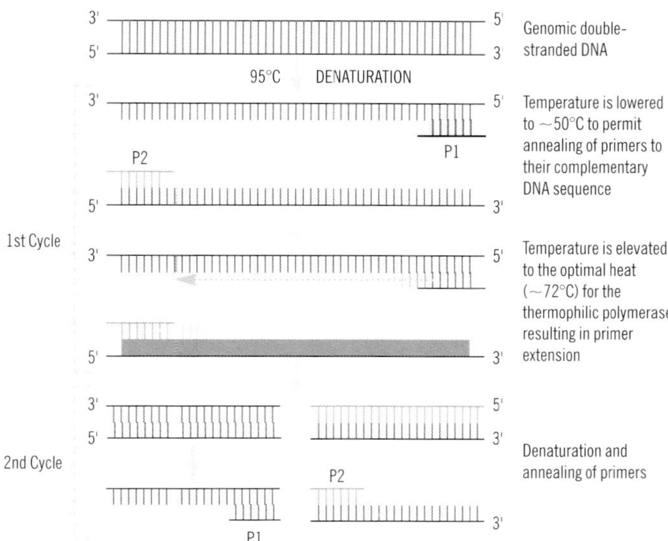

Figure 16. Schematic illustrating the technique of **polymerase chain reaction** (PCR).

reached, mainly for technical reasons. PCR has become a standard technique in molecular biology research as well as routine diagnostics.

Polymorphism May be applied to **phenotype** or **genotype**. The presence in a population of two or more distinct variants, such that the frequency of the rarest is at least 1% (more than can be explained by recurrent **mutation** alone). A **genetic locus** is polymorphic if its sequence exists in at least two forms in the population.

Premutation Any **DNA mutation** that has little, if any, phenotypic consequence but predisposes future generations to the development of full mutations with phenotypic sequelae. Particularly relevant in the analysis of diseases associated with **dynamic mutations**.

Proband (propositus) – index case The first individual to present with a disorder through which a **pedigree** can be ascertained.

Probe — General term for a molecule used to make a measurement. In molecular genetics, a probe is a piece of **DNA** or **RNA** that is labeled and used to detect its complementary sequence (e.g. **Southern blotting**).

Promoter region — The non-coding sequence upstream (5') of a **gene** where **RNA** polymerase binds. **Gene expression** is controlled by the promoter region both in terms of level and tissue specificity.

Protease — An enzyme that digests other proteins by cleaving them into small fragments; proteases may have broad specificity or only cleave a particular site on a protein or set of proteins.

Protease inhibitor — A chemical that can inhibit the activity of a **protease**. Most proteases have a corresponding specific protease inhibitor.

Proto-oncogene — A misleading term that refers to **genes** that are usually involved in signaling and cell development, and are often expressed in actively dividing cells. Certain **mutations** in such genes may result in malignant transformation, with the mutated genes being described as **oncogenes**. The term proto-oncogene is misleading because it implies that such genes were selected for by evolution in order that, upon mutation, cancers would result because of oncogenic activation. A similar problem arises with the term **tumor suppressor gene**.

Pseudogene — Near copies of true **genes**. Pseudogenes share sequence **homology** with true genes but are inactive as a result of multiple **mutations** over a long period of time.

Purine — A nitrogen-containing, double-ring, basic compound occurring in nucleic acids. The purines in **DNA** and **RNA** are **adenine** and **guanine**.

Pyrimidine — A nitrogen-containing, single-ring, basic compound that occurs in nucleic acids. The pyrimidines in **DNA** are **cytosine** and **thymine**, and cytosine and **uracil** in **RNA**.

Q

q — Long arm of a **chromosome** (see Figure 4).

R

Re-annealing — see **hybridization**

Recessive (traits, diseases) — Manifest only in homozygotes. For the **X chromosome**, recessivity applies to males who carry only one (mutant) **allele**. Females who carry **X-linked mutations** are generally heterozygotes and, barring unfortunate X-inactivation, do not manifest X-linked recessive **phenotypes**.

Reciprocal translocation — The exchange of material between two non-**homologous chromosomes**.

Recombination — The creation of new combinations of linked **genes** as a result of **crossing over** at **meiosis** (see Figure 6).

Recurrence risk — The chance that a genetic disease, already present in a member of a family, will recur in that family and affect another individual.

Restriction enzyme — **Endonuclease** that cleaves double-stranded (ds) **DNA** at specific sequences. For example, the enzyme *Bgl*II recognizes the sequence AGATCT, and cleaves after the first A on both strands. Most restriction endonucleases recognize sequences that are palindromic—the complementary sequence to AGATCT, read in the same orientation, is also AGATCT. The term 'restriction' refers to the function of these enzymes in nature. The organism that synthesizes a given restriction enzyme (e.g. *Bgl* I) does so in order to 'kill' foreign DNA—'restricting' the potential of foreign DNA that has become integrated to adversely affect the cell. The organism protects its own DNA from the restriction enzyme by simultaneously synthesizing a specific methylase that recognizes the same sequence and modifies one of the bases, such that the restriction enzyme is no longer able to cleave. Thus, for every restriction enzyme, it is likely that a corresponding methylase exists, although in practice only a relatively small number of these have been isolated.

Restriction fragment length polymorphism (RFLP) A restriction fragment is the length of **DNA** generated when DNA is cleaved by a **restriction enzyme**. Restriction fragment length varies when a **mutation** occurs within a restriction enzyme sequence. Most commonly the **polymorphism** is a single base substitution but it may also be a variation in length of a DNA sequence due to variable number tandem repeats (VNTRs). The analysis of the fragment lengths after DNA is cut by restriction enzymes is a valuable tool for establishing **familial** relationships and is often used in forensic analysis of blood, hair or semen (see Figure 11).

Restriction map A **DNA** sequence map, indicating the position of restriction sites.

Reverse genetics Identification of the causative **gene** for a disorder, based purely on molecular genetic techniques, when no knowledge of the function of the gene exists (the case for most genetic disorders).

Reverse transcriptase Catalyses the synthesis of **DNA** from a single-stranded **RNA** template. Contradicted the central dogma of genetics (DNA → RNA → protein) and earned its discoverers the Nobel Prize in 1975.

RNA (ribonucleic acid) RNA molecules differ from **DNA** molecules in that they contain a ribose sugar instead of deoxyribose. There are a variety of types of RNA (including **messenger RNA**, **transfer RNA** and ribosomal RNA) and they work together to transfer information from DNA to the protein-forming units of the cell.

Robertsonian translocation A **translocation** between two acrocentric **chromosomes**, resulting from centric fusion. The short arms and satellites (chromosome segments separated from the main body of the chromosome by a constriction and containing highly repetitive **DNA**) are lost.

S

Second hit hypothesis See **tumor suppressor gene**

Sex chromosomes Refers to the **X** and **Y chromosomes**. All normal individuals possess 46 chromosomes, of which 44 are **autosomes** and 2 are sex chromosomes. An individual's sex is determined by his/her complement of sex chromosomes. Essentially, the presence of a Y chromosome results in the male **phenotype**. Males have an X and a Y chromosome, while females possess two X chromosomes. The Y chromosome is small and contains relatively few **genes**, concerned almost exclusively with sex determination and/or sperm formation. By contrast, the X chromosome is a large chromosome that possesses many hundreds of genes.

Sex-limited trait A trait/disorder that is almost exclusively limited to one sex and often results from **mutations** in autosomal **genes**. A good example of a sex-limited trait is breast cancer. While males are affected by breast cancer, it is much less common (~1%) than in women. Females are more prone to breast cancer than males not only because they possess significantly more breast tissue but also because their hormonal milieu is significantly different. In many cases, early onset bilateral breast cancer is associated with mutations either in *BRCA1* or *BRCA2*, both autosomal genes. An example of a sex-limited trait in males is male pattern baldness which is extremely rare in pre-menopausal women. The inheritance of male pattern baldness is consistent with **autosomal dominant**, not **sex-linked dominant**, inheritance.

Sex-linked dominant See **X-linked dominant**

Sex-linked recessive See **X-linked recessive**

Sibship All the sibs in a family.

Silent mutation One that has no (apparent) phenotypic effect.

Single gene disorder	A disorder resulting from a **mutation** on one **gene**.
Somatic cell	Any cell of a multicellular organism not involved in the production of **gametes**.
Southern blot	**Hybridization** with a radio-labeled **RNA/DNA probe** to an immobilized DNA sequence (see Figure 17). Named after Ed Southern (currently Professor of Biochemistry at Oxford University, UK), the technique has spawned the nomenclature for other types of blot (**Northern blots** for RNA and **Western blots** for proteins).
Splicing	Removal of **introns** from precursor **RNA** to produce **messenger RNA**. The process involves recognition of intron-**exon** junctions and specific removal of intronic sequences, coupled with re-connection of the two strands of **DNA** that formerly flanked the intron.
Start codon	The AUG **codon** of **messenger RNA** recognized by the ribosome to begin protein production.
Stop codon	The **codons** UAA, UGA, or UAG on **messenger RNA** (mRNA) (see Table 2). Since no **transfer RNA** molecules exist that possess **anticodons** to these sequences, they cannot be translated. When they occur in frame on an mRNA molecule, protein synthesis stops and the ribosome releases the mRNA and the protein.

T

Telomere	End of a **chromosome**. The telomere is a specialized structure involved in replicating and stabilizing linear **DNA** molecules.
Teratogen	Any external agent/factor that increases the probability of congenital malformations. A teratogen may be a drug, whether prescribed or illicit, or an environmental effect, such as high temperature. The classical example is thalidomide, a drug originally prescribed for morning sickness, which resulted in very high rates of congenital malformation in exposed fetuses (especially limb defects).

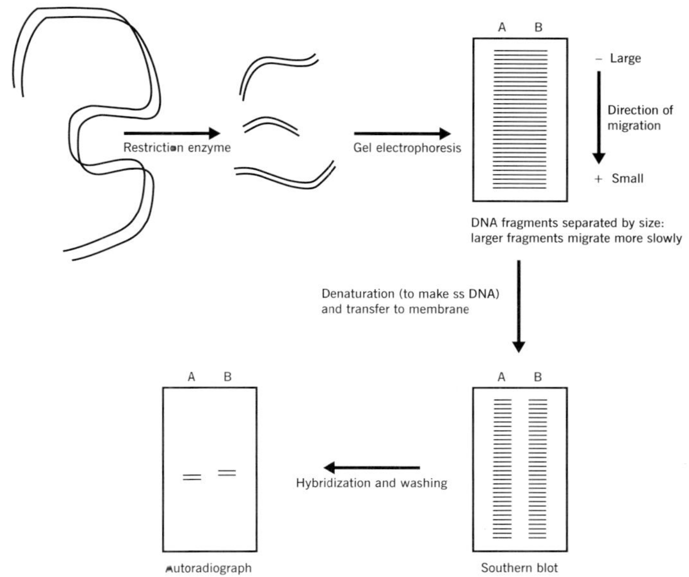

Figure 17. Southern blotting.

Termination codon See **stop codon**

Thymine (T) One of the bases making up **DNA** and **RNA** (pairs with **adenine**).

Transcription Synthesis of single-stranded **RNA** from a double-stranded **DNA** template (see Figure 18).

Transfer RNA (tRNA) An **RNA** molecule that possesses an **anticodon** sequence (complementary to the **codon** in mRNA) and the amino acid which that codon specifies. When the ribosome 'reads' the mRNA codon, the tRNA with the corresponding **anticodon** and amino acid is recruited for protein synthesis. The tRNA 'gives up' its amino acid to the production of the protein.

Translation Protein synthesis directed by a specific **messenger RNA** (mRNA), (see Figure 19). The information in mature mRNA is converted at

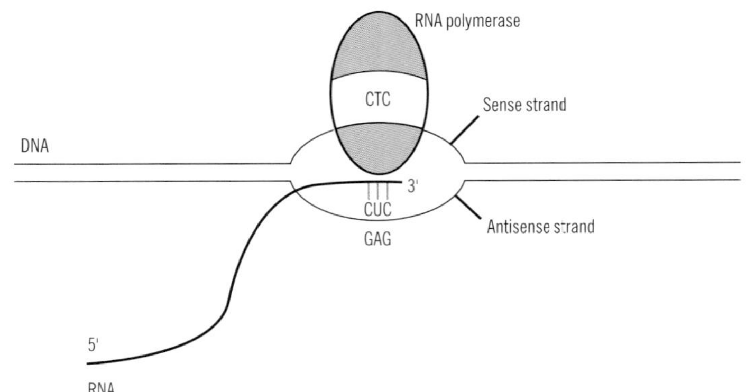

Figure 18. Schematic demonstrating the process of **transcription**. The sense strand has the sequence CTC (coding for leucine). **RNA** is generated by pairing with the antisense strand, which has the sequence GAG (the complement of CTC). The RNA produced is the complement of GAG, CUC (essentially the same as CTC, **uracil** replaces **thymine** in RNA).

the ribosome into the linear arrangement of amino acids that constitutes a protein. The mRNA consists of a series of trinucleotide sequences, known as **codons**. The **start codon** is AUG, which specifies that methionine should be inserted. For each codon, except for the **stop codons** that specify the end of translation, a **transfer RNA** (tRNA) molecule exists that possesses an **anticodon** sequence (complementary to the codon in mRNA) and the amino acid which that codon specifies. The process of translation results in the sequential addition of amino acids to the growing polypeptide chain. When translation is complete, the protein is released from the ribosome/mRNA complex and may then undergo post-translational modification, in addition to folding into its final, active, conformational shape.

Translocation

Exchange of chromosomal material between 2 or more non-**homologous chromosomes**. Translocations may be balanced or unbalanced. Unbalanced translocations are those that are observed in association with either a loss of genetic material, a gain, or both. As with other causes of **genomic** imbalance, there are usually

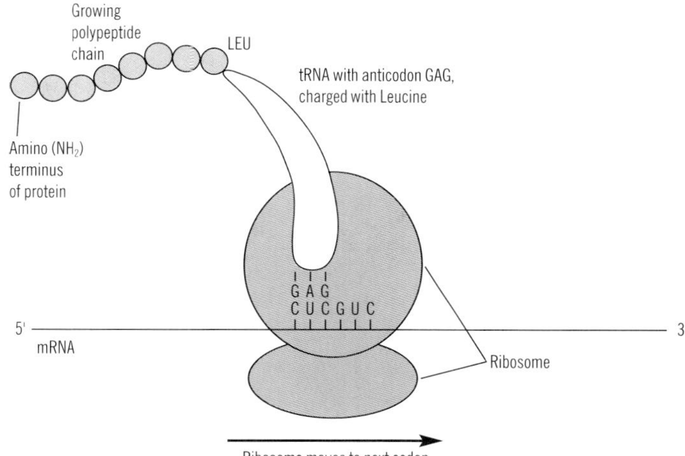

Figure 19. Schematic of the process of **translation**. **Messenger RNA** (mRNA) is translated at the ribosome into a growing polypeptide chain. For each **codon**, there is a **transfer RNA** molecule with the anticodon and the appropriate amino acid. Here, the amino acid leucine is shown being added to the polypeptide. The next codon is GUC, specifying valine. Translation happens in a 5' to 3' direction along the mRNA molecule. When the stop codon is reached, the polypeptide chain is released from the ribosome.

phenotypic consequences, in particular mental retardation. Balanced translocations are usually associated with a normal **phenotype** but increase the risk of genomic imbalance in offspring, with expected consequences (either severe phenotypes or lethality). Translocations are described by incorporating information about the chromosomes involved (usually but not always two) and the positions on the chromosomes at which the breaks have occurred. Thus t(11;X)(p13;q27.3) refers to an apparently balanced translocation involving chromosome 11 and X, in which the break on 11 is at 11p13 and the break on the X is at Xq27.3

Triplet repeats Tandem repeats in **DNA** that comprise many copies of a basic trinucleotide sequence. Of particular relevance to disorders associated with **dynamic mutations**, such as Huntington's chorea (HC). HC is associated with a pathological expansion of a CAG repeat within the coding region of the huntingtin **gene**. This repeat codes for a tract of polyglutamines in the resultant protein, and it is believed that the increase in length of the polyglutamine tract in affected individuals is toxic to cells, resulting in specific neuronal damage.

Trisomy

Possessing three copies of a particular **chromosome** instead of two.

Tumor suppressor genes

Genes that act to inhibit/control unrestrained growth as part of normal development. The terminology is misleading, implying that these genes function to inhibit tumor formation. The classical tumor suppressor gene is the Rb gene, which is inactivated in retinoblastoma. Unlike **oncogenes**, where a **mutation** at one **allele** is sufficient for malignant transformation in a cell (since mutations in oncogenes result in increased activity, which is unmitigated by the normal allele), both copies of a tumor suppressor gene must be inactivated in a cell for malignant transformation to proceed. Therefore, at the cellular level, tumor suppressor genes behave recessively. However, at the organismal level they behave as dominants, and an individual who possesses a mutation in only one Rb allele still has an extremely high probability of developing bilateral retinoblastomas.

The explanation for this phenomenon was first put forward by Knudson and has come to be known as the **Knudson hypothesis** (also known as the **second hit hypothesis**). An individual who has a germ-line mutation in one Rb allele (and the same argument may be applied to any tumor suppressor gene) will have the mutation in every cell in his/her body. It is believed that the rate of spontaneous somatic mutation (defined functionally, in terms of loss of function of that gene by whatever mechanism) is of the order of one in a million per gene per cell division. Given that there are many more than one million retinal cells in each eye, and many cell divisions involved in retinal development, the chance that the second (wild-type) Rb allele will suffer a somatic mutation is extremely high. In a cell that has acquired a 'second hit', there will now be no functional copies of the Rb gene, as the other allele is already mutated (germ-line mutation). Such a cell will have completely lost its ability to control cell growth and will eventually manifest as a retinoblastoma. The same mechanism occurs in many other tumors, the tissue affected being related to the tissue specificity of expression of the relevant tumor suppressor gene.

U

Unequal crossing over

Occurs between similar sequences on **chromosomes** that are not properly aligned. It is common where specific repeats are found and is the basis of many **microdeletion/microduplication** syndromes (see Figure 20).

Uniparental disomy (UPD)

In the vast majority of individuals, each **chromosome** of a pair is derived from a different parent. However, UPD occurs when an offspring receives both copies of a particular chromosome from only one of its parents. UPD of some chromosomes results in recognizable

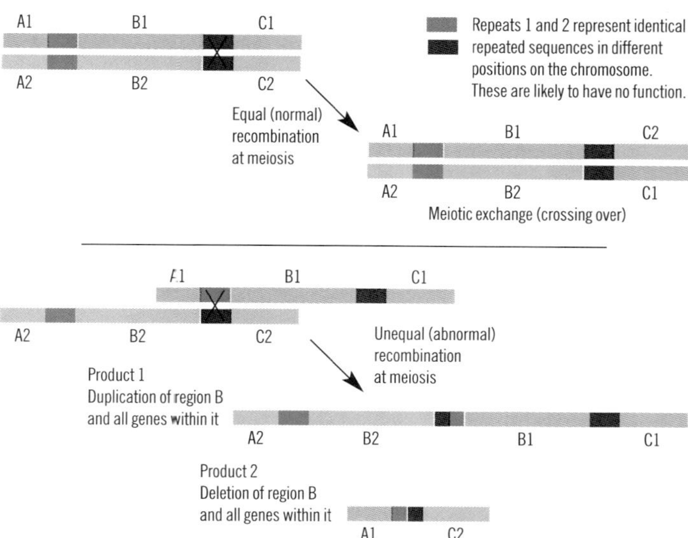

Figure 20. Schematic demonstrating (i) normal **homologous recombination** and (ii) homologous unequal recombination, resulting in a **deletion** and a duplication **chromosome**.

phenotypes whereas for other chromosomes there do not appear to be any phenotypic sequelae. One example of UPD is Prader-Willi syndrome (PWS), which can occur if an individual inherits both copies of chromosome 15 from their mother.

Uniparental heterodisomy — **Uniparental disomy** in which the two **homologues** inherited from the same parent are not identical. If the parent has **chromosomes** A,B the child will also have A,B.

Uniparental isodisomy — **Uniparental disomy** in which the two **homologues** inherited from the same parent are identical (i.e. duplicates). So, if the parent has **chromosomes** A,B then the child will have either A,A or B,B.

Uracil (U) — A nitrogenous base found in **RNA** but not in **DNA**, uracil is capable of forming a **base pair** with **adenine**.

V

Variable expressivity — Variable expression of a **phenotype**: not all-or-none (as is the case with **penetrance**). Individuals with identical **mutations** may manifest variable severity of symptoms, or symptoms that appear in one organ and not in another.

Variable number of tandem repeats (VNTR) — Certain **DNA** sequences possess tandem arrays of repeated sequences. Generally, the longer the array (i.e. the greater the number of copies of a given repeat), the more unstable the sequence, with a consequent wide variability between **alleles** (both within an individual and between individuals). Because of their variability, VNTRs are extremely useful for genetic studies as they allow for different alleles to be distinguished.

W

Western blot — Like a **Southern** or **Northern blot** but for proteins, using a labeled antibody as a probe.

X

X-autosome translocation **Translocation** between the **X chromosome** and an **autosome**.

X chromosome See **sex chromosomes**

X-chromosome inactivation See **Lyonisation**

X-linked Relating to the **X chromosome**/associated with **genes** on the X chromosome.

X-linked recessive (XLR) **X-linked** disorder in which the **phenotype** is manifest in **homozygous/hemizygous** individuals (see Figures 21a and 21b). In practice, it is hemizygous males that are affected by X-linked recessive disorders, such as Duchenne's muscular dystrophy (DMD). Females are rarely affected by XLR disorders, although a number of mechanisms have been described that predispose females to being affected, despite being **heterozygous**.

X-linked dominant (XLD) **X-linked** disorder that manifests in the heterozygote. XLD disorders result in manifestation of the **phenotype** in females and males (see Figure 22). However, because males are **hemizygous**, they are more severely affected as a rule. In some cases, the XLD disorder results in male lethality.

Y

Y chromosome See **sex chromosomes**

Z

Zippering A process by which complementary **DNA** strands that have annealed over a short length undergo rapid full annealing along their whole

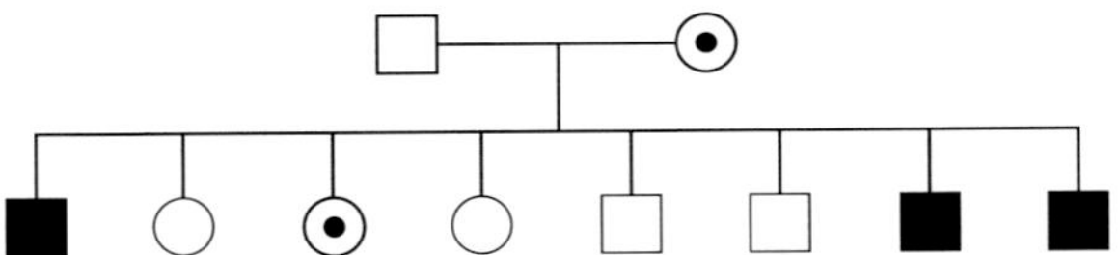

Figure 21a. X-linked recessive inheritance – A. Most X-linked disorders manifest recessively, in that **heterozygous** females (**carriers**) are unaffected and males, who are **hemizygous** (possess only one **X chromosome**) are affected. In this example, a carrier mother has transmitted the disorder to three of her sons. One of her daughters is also a carrier. On average, 50% of the male offspring of a carrier mother will be affected (having inherited the mutated X chromosome), and 50% will be unaffected. Similarly, 50% of daughters will be carriers and 50% will not be carriers. None of the female offspring will be affected but the carriers will carry the same risks to their offspring as their mother. The classical example of this type of inheritance is Duchenne's muscular dystrophy.

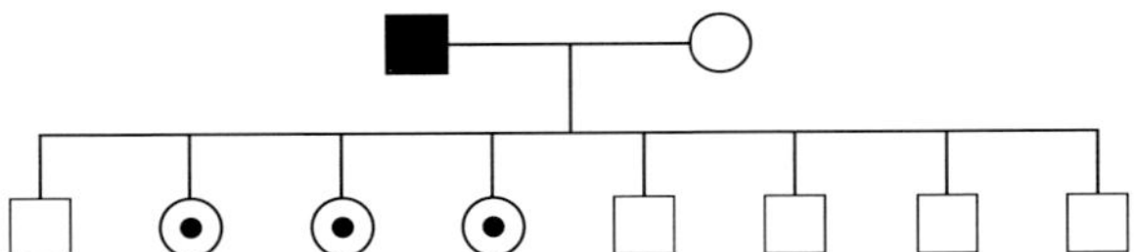

Figure 21b. X-linked recessive inheritance – B. In this example the father is affected. Because all his sons must have inherited their **Y chromosome** from him and their **X chromosome** from their normal mother, none will be affected. Since all his daughters must have inherited his X chromosome, all will be carriers but none affected. For this type of inheritance, it is clearly necessary that males reach reproductive age and are fertile—this is not the case with Duchenne's muscular dystrophy, which is usually fatal by the teenage years in boys. Emery-Dreifuss muscular dystrophy is a good example of this form of inheritance, as males are likely to live long enough to reproduce.

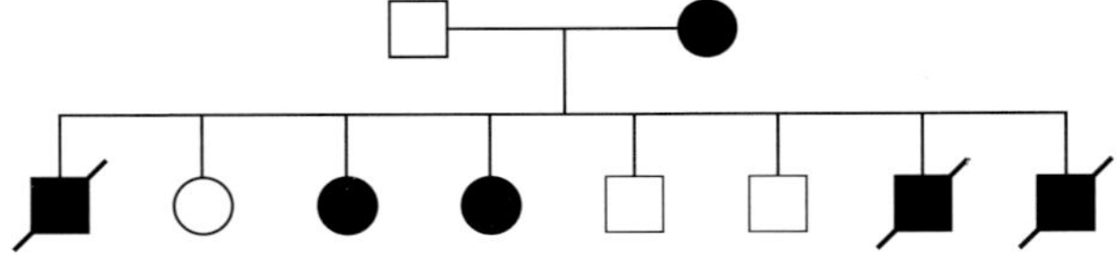

Figure 22. X-linked dominant inheritance. In X-linked dominant inheritance, the **heterozygous** female and hemizygous male are affected, however, the males are usually more severely affected than the females. In many cases, X-linked dominant disorders are lethal in males, resulting either in miscarriage or neonatal/infantile death. On average, 50% of all males of an affected mother will inherit the gene and be severely affected; 50% of males will be completely normal. Fifty percent of female offspring will have the same phenotype as their affected mother and the other 50% will be normal and carry no extra risk for their offspring. An example of this type of inheritance is incontinentia pigmenti, a disorder that is almost always lethal in males (males are usually lost during pregnancy).

length. DNA annealing is believed to occur in 2 main stages. A chance encounter of two strands that are complementary results in a short region of double stranded DNA which, if perfectly matched, stabilizes the two single strands so that further re-annealing of their specific sequences proceeds extremely rapidly. The initial stage is known as nucleation, while the second stage is called zippering.

Zygote — **Diploid** cell resulting from the union of male and female **haploid gametes**

13. Index

acanthosis nigricans **3**
acetylcholine receptor deficiency syndrome **156**
acetylcholinesterase deficiency syndrome **156**
achondrogenesis type IB **6**
achondroplasia **2–4**
acid alpha-glucosidase deficiency **152–3**
acid maltase deficiency **152–3**
acrochordons, and trichodiscomas **110**
ACT **42–3**
ACTA1 **164**
activated protein C resistance **97–8**
activation-induced cytidine deaminase **149**
ACVRLK1 **90**
ADA **136**
adenosine deaminase deficiency **136–7**
afibrinogenemia **102**
agammaglobulinemia
    Bruton type **146–7**
    Swiss type **138–9**
    X-linked **146–7**
AICDA **149**
airway disorders **14–41**
Aldrich syndrome **144–5**
alpha-1,4-glucosidase deficiency **152–3**
alpha$_1$-antichymotrypsin deficiency **42–3**
alpha$_1$-antitrypsin deficiency **44–7**
alpha-galactosidase A deficiency **55–6**
alveolar disorders **42–61**
alveolar proteinosis **51–2, 86**
amyloidosis, familial **83–4, 102**
amyotrophic lateral sclerosis **154–5**
anatomic defects **2–13**
Anderson-Fabry disease **55–6**
Angelman syndrome **180**
angiokeratoma corporis diffusum **55–6**
ankylosing spondylitis **78–80**
anti-elastase deficiency **44–7**
antithrombin III deficiency **99–100**
aortic aneurysm, without MFS **118**
AP3B **87**
ARSE **39**
arylsulfatase E activity **40**
aspirin-induced asthma **14–15**
asthma **14–19**
    aspirin-induced **14–15**
    nasal polyps **14–15**
AT3 **99**
ataxia-telangiectasia **122–3**
atelosteogenesis type 2 **5–6**
ATM **122–3**
ATP-binding cassette family **22**

bare lymphocyte syndrome, type I **132–3**
Bechterew's syndrome **78–80**
Becker muscular dystrophy **158–9**
beta$_2$-adrenergic receptor **17, 18**

beta-glucosidase deficiency **65–8**
beta-thalassemia **95**
Binder syndrome **26**
Birt-Hogg-Dube syndrome **110–11**
BLM **124**
blood disorders **90–109**
blood group A **49**
Bloom's syndrome **124–5**
BMPR2 **92**
bone morphogenetic protein receptor type 2 **92**
Bourneville's disease **186**
bronchiectasis
    Hermansky-Pudlak syndrome **87–8**
    Polynesian **32**
Bruton tyrosine kinase **146**
BTK **146**

campomelic dysplasia **7–8**
cathepsin K deficiency **36**
CBS **103**
CC16 **19**
CD3 deficiencies **143**
CD8 lymphopenia **142**
CD14 **19**
CD40LG **148**
central hypoventilation syndrome **170–2**
centronuclear myopathy **162–3**
ceramidase deficiency **62–4**
CFTR **22–3**
Charcot's disease **154–5**
chondrodysplasia punctata **38–40**
CHRNA1, *CHRNB1*, *CHRNE* **157**
chromosomal disorders **173**
chronic granulomatous disease **126–7**
chronic obstructive pulmonary disease **48–50**
chronic pneumonitis of infancy **85–6**
ciliary dyskinesia, primary **32–3**
Clara cell-specific 16 kD protein **19**
COL3A1 **112**
COLQ **156–7**
congenital alveolar proteinosis **51–2**
congenital central hypoventilation syndrome **170–2**
congenital myasthenic syndromes **156–7**
Conradi-Hünermann syndrome **38–40**
contractural arachnodactyly **118**
Crouzon's disease with acanthosis nigricans **3**
CSF2RB **51**
CTSK **36**
cutis laxa **53–4**
CYBA, *CYBB* **126–7**
cystathione beta-synthase **103**
cystic fibrosis **20–4**
cytochrome *P450IA1* **49, 178**
cytochrome *P450IIE* **178**

de la Chapelle dysplasia **5–6**

7-dehydrocholesterol reductase **11**
delta storage pool disease **87**
DHCR7 **11**
diastrophic dysplasia **6**
diaphragmatic spinal atrophy **167**
dibasicaminoaciduria II **57–8**
dilated cardiomyopathy, X-linked **159**
DKC1 **81**
DMD **158**
DMPK **160**
DNAI1 **32, 33**
DTDST **5**
Duchenne muscular dystrophy **158–9**
dynein axonemal intermediate chain 1 **32**
dysfibrinogenemia **101–2**
dysgammaglobulinemia type 1 **148–9**
dyskeratosis congenital **81–2**
dystrophia myotonica **160–1**
dystrophin **158**

EBP **39**
ectopia lentis **118**
EDN3 **170**
Ehlers-Danlos syndrome **112–13**
elastolysis **53–4**
endosteal hyperostosis **37**
endothelin 3 **170**
ENG (CD105) **90**

F2 **107**
F5 **97**
F13A **184**
Fabry's disease **55–6**
factor V Leiden **97–8, 108**
familial diseases
amyloidosis **83–4, 102**
aortic aneurysm without MFS **118**
atypical mycobacteriosis **130–1**
Hibernian fever **119–20**
infantile myasthenia syndrome **156–7**
interstitial lung disease **85–6**
Mediterranean fever **114–6, 120**
paroxysmal polyserositis **114–6**
periodic fever **119–20**
primary pulmonary hypertension **92–3**
Farber's lipogranulomatosis **62–4**
FBN1 **117**
FGFR3 **2**
fibrillin-1 protein **117**
fibrinogen, dysfibrinogenemia **101–2**
fibroblast growth factor family **2**
fibrofolliculomas, with trichodiscomas and acrochordons **110–1**

G2010A **107**
GAA **152**
galactocerebrosidase deficiency **69**

GALC **69**
Gaucher's disease **65–8**
GDNF **170**
GLA **55**
Gla protein, matrix **25**
glial cell line-derived neurotrophic factor **170**
globoid cell leukodystrophy **69–70**
glucocerebrosidase deficiency **65–8**
glutathione S-transferases **19, 49, 178**
glycogenoses **152–3**
GM1 gangliosidosis **73**
Golabi-Rosen syndrome **9–10**
GPC3 **9**
granulomatous disease, chronic **126–7**
GST **19**
GSTM1 **49, 178**

hamartin protein **186**
Happle syndrome **38–40**
HBB **94**
hemoglobin beta-globin **94**
heparan sulfate proteoglycan family **9**
heparin cofactor II deficiency **100**
hereditary dystopic lipidosis **55–6**
hereditary hemorrhagic telangiectasia **90–1**
hereditary polyserositis, recurrent **114–5**
Hermansky-Pudlak syndrome **87–8**
Hirschsprung's disease **170–1**
HLA **78, 183–4**
homocystinuria **103–4**
Hoyeraal-Hreidarsson syndrome **82**
HPS-1 **87**
Hunter's syndrome **30**
Hurler's syndrome **27–9**
Hurler-Scheie syndrome **27–9**
hyaline membrane disease **59–60**
hyper-IgE syndrome **128–9**
hyper-IgM syndrome, X-linked **148–9**
hyperhomocysteinemia **103–4**
hyperprothrombinemia **107–8**
hypochondroplasia **3**
hypoventilation syndrome, congenital central **170–2**

IDS **30**
IDUA **28**
iduronate 2-sulfatase deficiency **30–1**
iduronidase **28**
IFNGR1 deficiency **131**
IFNGR1, *IFNGR2* **130**
IgE receptor, beta chain **18**
IL-1alpha **184**
IL2RG **138**
IL-4 **17, 18**
IL-9 **19**
IL-12B **130**
IL12RB1 **130**

IL-13 **17, 18**
immotile ciliary syndrome **32–3**
immunodeficiencies **122–51**
  immunodeficiency 1 **146–7**
  immunodeficiency 3 **148–9**
  immunodeficiency 4 **138–9**
infantile subacute necrotizing encephalopathy **175–6**
infiltrative lung disorders **62–75**
interstitial lung disorders **77–88**
  familial interstitial lung disease **85–6**

JAK3 **138, 139**
Job syndrome **128–9**

Kartagener's syndrome **33**
Keutel syndrome **25–6**
Klinefelter's syndrome **173–4**
Krabbe's disease **69**

Leigh disease **175–6**
lethal acrodysgenital syndrome **11–2**
leukocyte mycobactericidal defect **130–1**
leukotriene C_4 synthase **14**
Liddle syndrome **35**
lipidosis, sphingomyelin **71–3**
lipogranulomatosis **62–4**
lipoprotein lipase deficiency **73**
Lou Gehrig's disease **154–5**
Louis—Bar syndrome **122–3**
LOX **53**
LTC4S **14**
lung cancer **177–8**
lysinuric protein intolerance **57–8**

major histocompatibility complex
  class I deficiency **132–3**
  class II deficiency **134–5**
Marfan's syndrome **117–8**
Marie-Strumpell spondylitis **78–80**
MASS phenotype **118**
matrix Gla protein **25**
MECP2 **181**
medullary thyroid carcinoma **171**
MEFV **114**
mEPHX **49**
MET **110**
methyl-CpG-binding protein-2 **181**
MGP **25**
MHC2TA **134**
microsomal epoxide hydrolase **49**
mineralocorticoid receptor **35**
mitochondrial myopathy, encephalopathy, lactic acidosis and stroke-like episodes (MELAS) **176**
Morquio syndrome **31**
MTATP6 **175**
MTM1 **162**
Muckle-Wells syndrome **84**

mucopolysaccharidosis **27–31**
Muenke coronal craniosynostosis **3**
multiple endocrine neoplasia types IIA, IIB **171**
muscular dystrophy (Becker and Duchenne) **158–9**
myasthenic syndromes, congenital **156–7**
mycobacteriosis, atypical **130–1**
myeloperoxidase **178**
MYF6 **163**
myoclonic epilepsy with ragged red fibers (MERRF) **176**
myotonic dystrophy **160–1**
myotubular myopathy **162–3**

NAD(P)H quinone oxidoreductase **178**
NCF1, *NCF2* **126**
NDUFS7, *NDUFS8* **175**
NDUFV1 **175**
NEB **164**
nemaline myopathy **164–5**
neonatal osseous dysplasia I **5–6**
neonatal respiratory distress syndrome **59–60, 86**
neuromuscular diseases **152–67**
Niemann-Pick disease, types A, B and C **71–5**
Nijmegen breakage syndrome **123**
NPC1 **74**
NQO1 **178**
NSAIDs, aspirin-induced asthma **14–15**

Omenn syndrome **140–1**
Ondine's curse **170–1**
Osler-Rendu-Weber disease **90–1**
osteogenesis imperfecta **37**
osteopetrosis **37**

p561ck defect **143**
PDHA1 **175**
periodic disease **114–5**
PI **45**
pleural disorders **110–20**
pneumonitis of infancy, chronic **85**
Polynesian bronchiectasis **32**
polyserositis, recurrent hereditary/familial paroxysmal **114–15**
Pompe's disease (infantile onset) **152–3**
Prader-Willi syndrome **179–80**
primary ciliary dyskinesia **32–3**
PROC **105**
PROS1 **105**
protease inhbitor 1 deficiency **44–7**
protein C/protein S deficiencies **105–6**
prothrombin gene mutation **107–8**
pseudohypoaldosteronism **34–5**
PSP-B **51**
pulmonary alveolar proteinosis **51–2, 86**
pulmonary hypertension, familial primary **92–3**
purine nucleoside phosphorylase deficiency **137**
pycnodysostosis **36–7**

RAG1, *RAG2* **140**
recombination-activating gene deficiency **140**
recurrent hereditary polyserositis **114–6**
respiratory distress syndrome **59–60**
RET **170–1**
reticular dysgenesia **141**
Rett syndrome **181–2**
RFX5 **134–5**
RFXANK **134–5**
RFXAP **134–5**
Rutledge lethal multiple congenital anomaly syndrome **11**

SADDAN dysplasia **3**
Sanfilippo syndrome **31**
saposin C **67**
sarcoidosis **183–5**
Scheie's syndrome **27–9**
sclerosteosis **37**
SCNN1A, 1B, 1G **34**
severe combined immunodeficiency
    due to adenosine deaminase deficiency **136–7**
    due to purine nucleoside phosphorylase deficiency **137**
    due to Zap-70 deficiency **142–3**
    T-negative, B-positive **138–9**
    T-negative, B-negative **140–1**
    V(D)J recombination defects **141**
SFTP2 **85**
Shprintzen-Goldberg syndrome **118**
sickle cell disease **94–6**
Simpson dysmorphia syndrome **9–10**
Simpson-Golabi-Behmel syndrome **9–10**
SLC7A7 **57**
SLO syndrome, types I and II **11–12**
slow channel syndrome **156–7**
Sly syndrome **31**
SMA I–III **166–7**
Smith-Lemli-Opitz syndrome **11–12**
SMN1, *SMN2* **166**
SMPD1 **72**
SNRPN **179–80**
SOD1 **154**
SOX9 **7**
SP-A1, *SP-A2* **59**
sphingomyelin lipidosis **71–3**
sphingomyelinase deficiency **71–3**
spinal muscular atrophy **166–7**
Steinert's disease **160–1**
SURF1 **175**
surfactant proteins **59–60**
Swiss type agammaglobulinemia **138–9**

TAP1, *TAP2* **132**
thalassemia **95**
thanatoporic dysplasia **3**
thymic epithelial hypoplasia **138–9**
TNF receptor-associated periodic syndrome **119–20**

TNF superfamily **148**
TNF alpha **19, 49**
TNF beta **184**
TNFRSF1A **119**
TPM3 **164**
transcription factors, SRY family **7**
transforming growth factor receptor superfamily **90, 92**
transporter associated with antigen processing **132**
transthyretin **83**
TRAPS (TNF receptor-associated periodic syndrome) **119–20**
trichodiscomas, and acrochordons **110**
TSC1, *TSC2* **186**
TTR **83**
tuberin **186**
tuberous sclerosis **186–8**

vas deferens, absence **24**
vascular disorders **90–108**
VHL **110**
vitamn D binding protein (VDBP) **49**

Waardenburg-Shah syndrome **171**
WASP **144**
Wiskott-Aldrich syndrome **144–5**
Wolman disease **73**

X-linked disorders
- agammaglobulinemia **146–7**
- chondrodysplasia punctata **38–40**
- dilated cardiomyopathy **159**
- hyper-IgM syndrome **148–9**
- Klinefelter's syndrome **173–4**

ZAP70 **142**
Zinsser-Cole-Engman syndrome **81–2**